How to Help Your Doctor Help You

A Guide for Men and Women to Manage Health Proactively

Bonita Coe MD, MBA

13TH & JOAN

For permission requests, write to the publisher, addressed "Attention: Permissions Coordinator," 205 N. Michigan Avenue, Suite #810, Chicago, IL 60601. 13th & Joan books may be purchased for educational, business or sales promotional use. For information, please email the Sales Department at sales@13thandjoan.com.

Printed in the U. S. A.

First Printing, October 2024.

Library of Congress Cataloging-in-Publication Data has been applied for.

ISBN: 978-1-961863-99-6

Every patient that I have ever taken care of has poured into me what is poured onto the pages of this book.

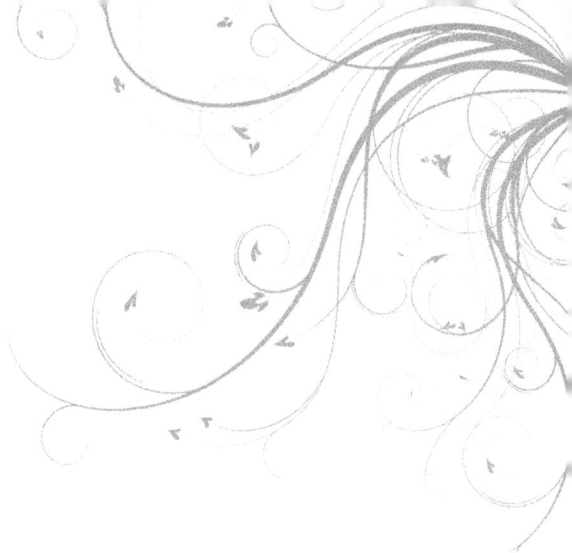

Contents

BE AN ACTIVE PARTICIPANT IN YOUR HEALTH: BEING HEALTHY AND FIT IS A LIFESTYLE

MAINTENANCE OF HEALTH

THE PAINLESS NATURE OF DIABETES, HIGH BLOOD PRESSURE, AND HIGH CHOLESTEROL

GETTING TO YOUR WEIGHT LOSS GOAL

YOUR MENTAL HEALTH CONTROLS YOUR PHYSICAL HEALTH

Introduction

THE GOAL OF THIS BOOK IS TO PROVIDE EVERYDAY individuals a single comprehensive resource, that shares the wisdom and practical tips I've gained from my clinical practice, focusing on health, mental health, and overall wellness. My philosophy and unique approach to caring for people is informed by the many self-observations that I have accumulated from my patients over the years. This book aims to simplify the reader's approach to health, making it feel less daunting and removing the fear or hesitation that often leads to avoiding medical advice and neglecting one's well-being. This book is invaluable to people who have doctors but are not getting what they want out of their health care interactions.

According to the May 16, 2023 Time Magazine article, more than 70% of Americans feel that our healthcare system is failing to meet their needs in some way (https://time.com/6279937/us-health-care-system-attitudes/). An April 24, 2024 U.S. News and World Report survey documented several reasons why many Americans won't go to the doctor including not liking to go to the doctor (25%) and having negative experiences with medical care in the past (10%). (https://health. usnews.com/health-care/top-doctors/articles/primary-care-experiences-survey-report#:~:text=25%25%20said%20they%20 don't,others%20during%20a%20PCP%20visit).

We all want to live fulfilling lives with minimal interruption from medical conditions or illnesses. With so much information readily available at our fingertips, I've long stopped being surprised by how little people actually know about promoting and maintaining their long-term health. There is so much information that people have access to, however it is hard for people to sift through the noise and focus on what is important and what actually makes a difference in health and wellness. Despite the amount of money that we spend on healthcare in this country, our collective health should be much better than what it is. A report from The Commonwealth Fund shows that "the United States spends more on healthcare than any other high-income country but still has the lowest life expectancy at birth and the highest rate of people with multiple chronic diseases." (https://www. cnn.com/2023/01/31/health/us-health-care-spending-global-perspective/index.html) In addition, this book can be a great supplement for people who need impactful information about promoting their health, as it explains the subject matter with details that may not be provided by their own doctors, due to lack of access and time constraints during doctor visits. Much has been written in the popular press and research journals about the crisis of the shortage of primary care physicians in this country, for example, the October 25, 2024 American Medical Association's president's address sounding the alarm about the crisis (https:// www.ama-assn.org/press-center/press-releases/ama-president-sounds-alarm-national-physician-shortage). People are finding it increasingly difficult to secure a primary care physician, get an appointment within a reasonable timeframe, and have enough time with their doctor to address all their medical concerns and questions.

As a practicing primary physician, I see too many adult patients that are struggling with burgeoning chronic medical conditions and illnesses. They are frustrated and overwhelmed with trying to live busy lives and maintain the quality of life that they deserve. Maintaining and advocating for one's health is not easy, but it can be done. This book reflects how I care for my patients every day and is written with the goal of helping more people take charge of their own health. I decided to write it to reach a broader audience and provide practical advice on becoming a stronger advocate for personal well-being. I want to share the wisdom and the pearls that my patients have given me that I pass on to other patients every day as well as my distinct way of approaching health and wellness that the reader can incorporate in their lives in a meaningful and impactful way. So many of my patients have asked me over the years, "Why has no one told me this before?" when I discuss their medical issues and formulate a management plan for their health that is working, when nothing has worked before.

The book gives detailed information about how to proactively help you care for yourself and also help your physician/provider care for you in a more substantial way. There are so many things that patients can do to promote and maintain health and improve ill-health. I spend a good portion of the book focusing on advice that I have gathered about making life choices that affect current and future health. This advice has been gleaned from listening to the life stories and experiences of my many patients, as I work with them over time. In addition, I focus on practical ways to make healthy choices in life with respect to eating, prevention and management of chronic diseases and conditions and keeping track of mental health status. The advice contained in these pages stems from listening to the life stories and experiences of many patients throughout my career as an Internal Medicine physician. I give practical ways to make healthy choices in life with respect to eating, prevention and management of chronic diseases and conditions and keeping track of your mental health status.

About fifteen years ago, I developed the habit of jotting down memorable, insightful, and practical things my patients said—things I wanted to remember and share with others in future sessions. I started with a small spiral notebook that I would keep in my white coat pocket that initially was used for equations and calculations that I used often in patient care. Keeping a small notebook with frequently needed calculations was a habit that I started in medical school and residency. I would write down the patients' statements and sayings on a sticky note and then transfer them to the pocket notebook when I got a chance.

I don't remember when I first said to myself, "I need to write a book with these," but I do remember that at the time I said it, in my mind, it was going to be a long way off. I did realize that what I was writing down was wisdom from my patients that I could not learn in medical school or in residency. The wisdom that I was collecting is the type of wisdom that can only be gathered from getting to know patients and taking care of people over time.

As I progressed with my career and practice, I found that I began to have more patient quips and quotes in the notebook than equations. I either didn't need to use the equations anymore in my current practice, the equations were obsolete, or I could access the equations more in the electronic medical record (EMR) clinical reference resources and online clinical databases as I began to do away with keeping things written on paper. In 2016 or

2017, I put all of the quips and quotes from my notebook, the multi-colored sticky notes that were stuck together, and notes in my phone note section for this purpose into a Microsoft Word document.

I began to organize the notes by topic and started a document that for the first time started to look like a book with chapters. I said to myself, "I think I should start this book I keep telling myself about." I then began to expand on each "chapter" by using my clinical experience of taking care of patients to explain the common issues encountered by my patients. Active listening to patients helped me hone my clinical skills such that I have developed a distinctive way of taking care of patients that helps them get improvement of their health when they have not been satisfied with the care that they have been receiving from previous doctors. Paying attention to what my patients communicate has propelled me to be a distinguished clinician, diagnostician, counselor and advocate for the people that I care for.

I realized that the advice that I give to my patients wasn't just effective because I was a good clinician, but also that I used what I learned from my patients to help the next patient (and even sometimes myself).

Many of the chapter titles in this book are inspired by my patients' quotes, with some chapters beginning by explaining the context of the health concern they were addressing. I weave these patient experiences into the narrative, incorporating the essential knowledge I wish my patients came prepared with when engaging in their care. This would allow me to take care of them more effectively. I've documented all the key questions I ask new patients—information I believe every adult should know. Additionally, I've included healthy eating tips and weight loss success strategies shared by my patients.

An early book title I considered was "What My Patients Have Taught Me" or "Pearls from My Patients," as I looked over all of the clever things my patients taught me over the years.

In 2019 or 2020, I started to expand the project to include impressions from patient interactions that day. I would dictate into the document on my cell phone in the car while driving home as the interaction was fresh in my mind. I then started to dictate new chapters about topics to record my thoughts related to discussions with patients that day that I wanted to remember and share with other patients. I came up with the final title "How to Help Your Doctor Help You" when I started to add topics to share in the soon-to-be book when I would be dictating (more like venting to my phone) about things I wish they already knew so I could more effectively take care of them. But, then again... how would they know? I started dictating things that I ask all new patients every day that I wished all my new patients came to the office with on the first visit (for example, medical records, medication list, blood pressure, and blood pressure readings). Over the years, I have had so many patients respond to my advice, "I didn't know to do that," "Nobody ever told me that," when I give advice about healthy eating, ask medical history questions and give advice about all kinds of practical issues and ways to improve medical issues, mental health and overall well-being. So many patients tell me they wish the advice I had given them had been shared many years before.

This book tells people, in clear terms, full of lists, charts and checklists, about how to keep up with mental and physical health, such that they can actually help their doctor take better care of them and become an engaged and informed advocate for their own health. My advice can help improve health, control and reverse many chronic medical illnesses and conditions and can even decrease or eliminate the need for prescription medications. I write down healthy eating tips, weight loss success strategies from patients and use the advice to help future patients.

The first three sections of the book are a collection of my thoughts, much of which has been inspired by my patients, about how to begin to transform your thinking about what is health and wellness and how you can make proactive and deliberate choices to promote the best outcome possible for your health for the rest of your life. In these sections, I give specific recommendations about how to actively participate in your healthcare so that your doctor can make the best recommendations possible for you. I encourage you to become a partner with your doctor to get a comprehensive assessment of your health, focusing on the aspects of any evaluation that you have with your doctor that will make a difference in your wellness and well-being in the future. I provide detailed guidance on advocating for your own healthcare while also assisting your doctor in providing better care for you. Since I take care of adults from early adult life to the end of life, I wrote "Advice for the Decades" to provide the reader with an overview of medical and life issues that people experience over time that impact their health and ability to attend to and maintain health, fitness, and well-being. Much of this information is peppered with the wealth of wisdom and reflection on their lives that my older patients gave often. I incorporated preventive health recommendations and healthy eating recommendations that I give to patients every day. It will help you to see these items in a succinct version so that you can begin to have a more organized approach to how you eat and proactively plan how you want to reach your health care goals. Patients frequently tell me they've never encountered information presented in a way that allows them to fully grasp it and start making lifestyle changes to reach their health goals.

The next two sections are meant to impart drilled down information about what you can do to prevent or manage diabetes, high blood pressure, high cholesterol, and/or obesity, which are four conditions that are very important to be identified and addressed. These four conditions are significant contributors to heart and vascular disease in this country.

The next section of this book takes a deep dive into how much mental health plays a role in physical health and overall well-being. I relied heavily on my patients' wisdom and life experiences they have told me about to compile this section about the pitfalls in life that can derail your health. I end the book with some specific pearls and caveats for the female patient regarding bladder function and the intersectionality between mental health, women's health, and vaginal function.

In the Epilogue, I offer my thoughts about healthcare delivery from a national perspective. After taking care of patients in our healthcare "system" for the last twenty years, I have developed a few opinions about how we need to improve healthcare delivery in this country.

I added an Appendix to this book because I could not write a book like this without imparting information about Advanced Directives and end of life considerations that we all need to think about in advance, regardless of age. Even younger adults should think about end-of-life issues, as young adults often have acute illness and injury, where there is no time to discuss your wishes in the event, if even temporarily, you cannot make medical decisions for yourself. This information did not exactly flow with the premise of the book, but it certainly is an extremely important part of making proactive decisions about your health. I began the bulk of the compilation and the writing of this book in 2020, and I felt compelled to add my thoughts in the Appendix about my experiences with the incorporation of the significant amount of delivery of healthcare with telemedicine in this country that began with the onset and continuation of the COVID 19 pandemic.

In addition, the Appendix contains all of the website references that are in the book by chapter with the corresponding QR codes to make accessing the resources easy.

I hope you'll use this book to embrace the various concepts and strategies discussed, empowering yourself to improve your health and the well-being of your family.

Always consult with a qualified and licensed physician or other medical care provider, and follow their advice without delay regardless of anything read in this book.

External (outbound) links in the references to other websites or educational material are followed at your own risk. Under no circumstances is the author responsible for the claims of third-party websites or educational providers.

PATIENT VIGNETTE DISCLAIMER

The patient vignettes that are included in this book are from actual patients that I have taken care of at some point in my career, however aspects of the vignettes have been changed to make sure that no patient can be identified by the clinical information provided. In some cases, the examples are a combination of patients that had similar clinical presentations. I included these examples throughout the book to illustrate real life examples of the successes and challenges that are common in an everyday primary care practice.

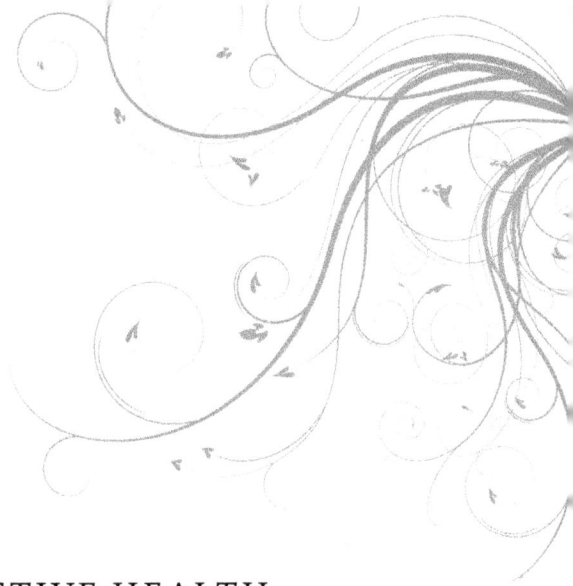

PROACTIVE HEALTH

Tomorrow belongs to people who prepare for it today.
African Proverb

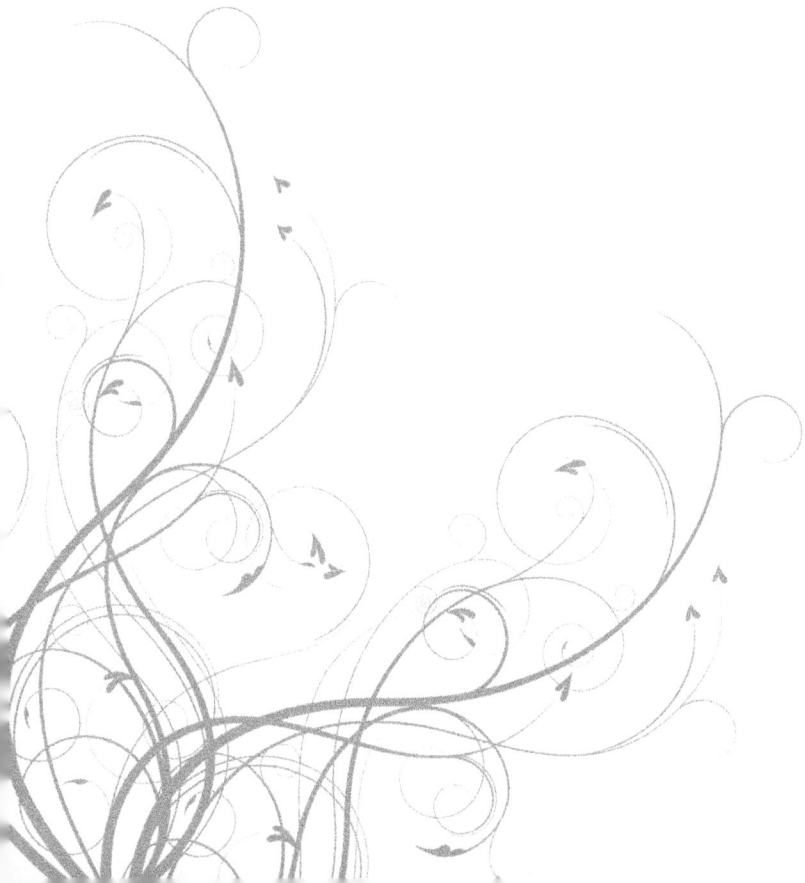

1

"I Am Not Claiming It." If You Don't Claim It, It May Claim You

WE'VE ALL HAD THE EXPERIENCE OF SAYING SOMETHING aloud or having a thought and soon thereafter, what we said or thought about *actually happened*. In addition, many of us have grown up with (at home and with formal spiritual teachings) the concept of not speaking or "claiming" negative things to stay on a positive course in life. This concept of not saying or thinking negative things goes a long way to maintaining a positive environment, keeping us spiritually grounded and keeping good things and experiences coming our way.

Unfortunately, a doctor visit can be one of those experiences in life where the conversation may include undesirable, unwelcomed, and unfavorable information. The visit can cause unease and apprehension about medical issues that you may have that are going to affect your life. It becomes even more anxiety producing as one gets older and/or when friends and family start to be diagnosed with adverse medical conditions. In addition, the readily available access to information (including misinformation) on the internet has heightened awareness about medical illness, conditions, and preventive health, but also raised the level of anxiety about developing a medical illness. Sometimes anxiety can lead to staying at a level of comfort and denial about a medical condition. However, it is my experience that in the long run, it is better to be proactive with your health. It is better to prevent medical conditions from starting in the first place and/or address medical conditions so they do not get worse or stay uncontrolled.

A lot of patients tell me they choose not to "claim" a medical issue that I have just told them about, where they are reluctant to accept a new diagnosis that has been identified. It is typically a serious or chronic disease that does not have a cure but needs to be managed with or without medication indefinitely. Many of these medical conditions have mild symptoms or no symptoms at all but have been identified by doing recommended preventive health screenings.

Many patients who are fearful about a medical condition communicate to me their preference to rely on their faith to see them through. Instead, I encourage patients to consider relying on their faith to proceed with the recommended evaluation, treatment, or lifestyle modification so the medical problem or potential medical problem can be appropriately addressed. In addition, I encourage patients to use their faith to engage in the discussion about their health and "speak" and "think" better health into existence going forward.

Most commonly, the chronic diseases that people are reluctant to accept are asthma, diabetes, hypertension, and high cholesterol. These are very important conditions to identify and manage because they are big drivers of the cardiovascular disease burden that people have in this country. Chronic diseases are those that are not going to cause death soon, but the progression of the condition can lead to symptoms that worsen over time, undesirable complications, and a decline in quality of life.

When the new diagnosis is being presented, I find it helpful to review with a patient how I arrived at the diagnosis. For issues like diabetes, high cholesterol, and high blood pressure, it is simply a blood pressure check taken in the office or a defining blood test result number that the patient has reached. For other conditions, the diagnosis may be defined by the person's symptoms and diagnostic testing.

It is often hard to accept a diagnosis that is not causing any symptoms. I am often presenting undesirable information after I have reviewed their previous medical records, especially with a new patient. Often, patients have received diagnoses from previous doctors or specialists without being informed. Then I am put in the awkward position of explaining a diagnosis or asymptomatic medical condition to a patient, despite the diagnosis already being found per documentation in previous records.

It often takes time to get the person to accept the diagnosis enough to move them to the point where we can take steps to manage and treat the condition. For chronic conditions like high blood pressure, diabetes, and high cholesterol, the initial recommendation does not necessarily include taking medication indefinitely. For many, it means starting with making lifestyle changes and modifications, including improving eating habits and getting regular exercise. For others, it may mean taking medications and even seeing a specialist.

Unfortunately for many people, these illnesses may have a strong genetic component and may not be able to be eliminated entirely by making changes in food choices and getting regular exercise. However, the amount and dose of medication that may need to be taken can be decreased by making the recommended lifestyle changes. These changes need to be continued indefinitely. In fact, many people can reverse or improve many medical conditions by being conscious of the food they eat and getting regular exercise.

Even degenerative joint conditions, like what is commonly known as arthritis (osteoarthritis, not to be confused with osteoporosis), can be improved with adjusted eating habits and losing weight. Many people with degenerative, inflammatory, and /or autoimmune joint and muscle conditions (lupus, rheumatoid arthritis, etc.) feel better by choosing more plant-based foods and avoiding animal products like beef, lamb, milk, and cheese from a cow.

Having uncontrolled high blood pressure, uncontrolled diabetes, and high cholesterol increases the cardiovascular risk like heart attack, stroke, kidney failure, being on dialysis, blindness, peripheral vascular disease (blocked arteries/poor circulation in the legs and feet), and lower extremity amputations and eye disease leading to blindness, to name a few. Poor management of chronic conditions often leads to having to take more medications and the need to see more specialists as the condition worsens.

Many people still die from asthma too often in this country. For me, the management of chronic asthma has a particular meaning because of an experience I had with a patient during residency.

It was during an emergency department rotation one Saturday that a patient was driven to the emergency department (ED) by her family because she was having an asthma attack and was not breathing well. They drove her directly to the ED ambulance entry door and she was immediately taken from the car on a stretcher because she could not walk by herself. Her eyes were closed, and she was not moving. By the time we got her into the ED, she was barely breathing. One family member told us she had asthma, suddenly had asthma symptoms at home, and that she had not been taking her asthma medications. She was immediately intubated and placed on a ventilator (machine that takes over control of breathing). Her airways were so tight that even the ventilator machine could not open her airways. She passed away in the ED. I will never forget that experience. This experience has shaped the way I "push" my patients to establish good habits with their chronic disease management. It can really be a matter of life and death.

The bottom line is this: Denying the existence of a condition and avoiding management of a condition is not the solution. Leaving medical conditions uncontrolled can lead to terrible consequences. These negative outcomes can be avoided by following the instructions from your doctor regarding how you should be eating, doing home self-monitoring (checking blood pressure and blood sugar at home), taking medication as prescribed, and doing regular follow up visits with your doctor to assess the status of your condition as recommended.

Choices Based on Fear

$\mathcal{P}$ EOPLE OFTEN AVOID COMING TO THE DOCTOR BECAUSE of fear of the unknown. In my experience, people avoid or delay seeking care for several reasons:

- They are apprehensive about the status of a known diagnosis or condition, possible diagnosis, or the fear the new symptoms could be something very serious.
- People also fear the anticipated process that may be needed to arrive at a diagnosis and/or fear the subsequent treatment.
- People also decline things like preventive health screenings (colonoscopies, mammograms, Pap tests, bone density tests, screening blood tests, sexually transmitted disease screening, screening for high cholesterol and diabetes blood tests) and vaccinations because of fear of the procedure and the condition that the procedure will find (hopefully early) or prevent.

I had a patient who was very fearful of getting a colonoscopy screening. The purpose of getting a colonoscopy is to look at the large intestine to find and remove pre-cancerous areas, called polyps, that can turn into colon cancer if left in place. At the time of our first discussion about colon cancer screening, he was ten years past the age when colon cancer screening was recommended to be started. His mother and younger sister were also my patients, and they could not convince him to get a colonoscopy either. The reason why it was particularly important for him to get a colonoscopy was because his father had colon cancer. Having a parent that had colon cancer made it even more critical for him to do regular colon cancer screening. His sister got her colonoscopy, and it was normal. His other siblings, who were not my patients, got their colonoscopies done and they were all normal, which he shared with me one visit when we discussed it again. As time went on, he came one day to see me with abdominal symptoms 2-3 years after we first discussed that he needed to get a colonoscopy.

Because he was having symptoms, a colonoscopy was definitely part of the workup that would be needed to evaluate his abdominal concerns. Finally, he agreed to get the colonoscopy. Unfortunately, colon cancer was present, and he ultimately needed to have surgery to remove the part of the colon that was cancerous. He and his family were relieved it had not spread such that he didn't also need chemotherapy.

Before undergoing any procedure or test, including a simple blood test, it's advisable to discuss the reasons with your doctor or at least receive written information explaining why the test is recommended. The risk and benefit of getting the test or procedure should also be reviewed and the possible or anticipated result should also be considered. In addition, if the next step following an abnormal result is undesired (more testing, a biopsy, surgery, chemotherapy, radiation, etc.), then it should be considered that the initial test being discussed should not be done at all. Once you know about an abnormal test result, it is hard to go back to the frame of mind of when you didn't know that the abnormality existed.

People often look up symptoms and conditions on the Internet and see the worst-case scenarios, instead of consulting with a medical professional for their questions and concerns. People get information from social media, friends, and family who often give misinformation and bad advice, even though it may be well-intentioned. The information obtained from the Internet may be correct but may not apply to you as an individual. In addition, the internet has alarming pictures of medical conditions that cannot be verified as an image of the condition being portrayed. I find that people have more fear and anxiety after looking up symptoms and medical conditions on the internet, and it causes more problems than it solves.

Fear often comes from lack of knowledge and unfamiliarity. Often a person's fears can be addressed by giving information in terms the person can understand, then a better-informed decision can be made. Even if a person ultimately chooses not to do a test, it can be said that the person has made the decision based on knowledge and not just emotion.

3

Don't Ignore Chest and Abdominal Pain, Trouble Breathing, or Seeing Blood

*T*HERE ARE CERTAIN SYMPTOMS THAT ABSOLUTELY SHOULD NOT be ignored because doing so can lead to serious complications, morbidity, and mortality. It's always a good decision to have ANY symptom(s), especially any new symptom(s), evaluated for which there is no reasonable explanation.

These are the 4 general categories of symptoms that people ignore or delay seeking care about that can have devastating consequences if disregarded.

CHEST PAIN

Several causes of chest pain can occur in people, regardless of age, that can have devastating consequences if immediate medical attention is not sought. This is not an exhaustive list, however, the most serious causes are heart attack, pulmonary embolism (blood clots in lungs), aortic dissection (splitting of the lining of the large artery that comes from the heart to give blood to the rest of the body) and asthma. Asthma symptoms in adults can be a persistent cough and chest pain and is not always an obvious symptom, like trouble breathing. No matter how old you are, you should always seek medical care immediately for chest pain. I have had many patients who have had chest pain for hours to months without seeking care. They often try home treatments in an effort to try to figure out the cause of their symptoms instead of seeking medical attention.

I remember a patient in his 40s who was having new chest pain that was occurring off and on for 2-3 weeks. The pain was significant enough to him that after 2-3 weeks of the symptom, he mentioned it to his wife. He did not have a primary care doctor. His wife kept insisting that he see a doctor about the chest pain, and he called my office and scheduled a new patient appointment to establish care two days later. He did not mention his chest pain when he was asked the reason for his visit.

It became clear, as the visit progressed, that his main concern was his chest pain. He reported that his wife was more concerned about it than he was because he thought he was too young to have a serious health problem and he had no previous medical problems. He was not taking any medication and had never smoked tobacco and was not overweight. With direct questioning, I was able to find out he was having chest pain, mostly with walking. After completing his visit, I discussed my concern that the cause of his chest symptom could be coming from his heart not getting enough blood due to having a blocked artery in the heart (angina). I remember the details of this, because it was a Friday afternoon. If it had been earlier in the week, I could have arranged for him to get a stress test (a heart test to safely "stress" the heart to see if there is evidence of the heart not getting enough blood from blocked arteries that supply blood to the heart). But since this was a Friday afternoon, I decided that going to the ER would be the best advice, since an outpatient stress test could not possibly be arranged until at least Monday. If he had blocked heart arteries, waiting two more days for testing could be two days too late.

As I suspected, he immediately told me he did not want to go to the ER to have his symptoms evaluated. I decided to involve his wife in the conversation to help. After she was called, I explained the situation to her, and she was able to convince him to go to the ER four blocks away from my office. Once there, he was evaluated by a heart specialist (cardiologist). He was admitted to the hospital and had a cardiac catheterization (a diagnostic procedure to directly look at the blood flow in the arteries that give blood to the heart) on Saturday morning. He had a blockage in 2 of the 3 main arteries that give blood to the heart and had stents (small devices placed in the artery to open blockages) placed.

I saw him at his follow-up visit two weeks later, and he and his wife were very grateful that I pushed him to go to the ER immediately. In the hospital, he was educated about low-fat eating and was prescribed several medications by the cardiologist that help to keep blocked arteries open and prevent heart attacks. He told me the cardiologist told him that he was at very high risk of having a heart attack very soon, if he had not sought medical attention for his symptoms. The patient was very surprised that he had blocked heart arteries (coronary artery disease) and that this could happen in someone that did not have any other previously diagnosed medical conditions. He had further testing, and it was discovered he did not have high blood pressure or diabetes, but was found to have high cholesterol. Having high cholesterol is a significant risk factor for coronary artery disease, heart attacks and strokes.

ABDOMINAL PAIN

There are a myriad of causes for pain in the abdominal area and the list of possibilities depends on many factors your doctor can help sort out. It is not recommended that a person try to "figure out" the cause because there are so many possibilities that can have severe consequences. Unfortunately, time lost trying to self-diagnose may be the difference between life and death. Seeking medical attention early can help you find serious causes and prevent possible complications. The most important thing about having abdominal pain is finding out if the cause is due to a condition that has to be emergently addressed. Critical or life-threatening causes of abdominal pain don't have to be severe to still be dangerous, if left untreated. In addition, abdominal symptoms that have been going on for weeks to months can be just as serious as symptoms that just started within hours.

I had a patient with abdominal pain that had been going on for many months. She described it as a "gnawing" intermittent pain in the upper part of her abdomen, but she didn't have any other symptoms and she was able to carry on with her daily activities. She made an appointment one day to get my opinion because it was not going away despite her trial of various over the counter treatments and home remedies. Outpatient evaluation revealed that she had an inflamed gallbladder from gallstones, which had to be removed because her gallbladder was infected.

In the abdomen, the body has the ability to protect itself from serious processes that are going on but cannot maintain that state indefinitely. Serious conditions leading to abdominal infection or bleeding are common causes of abdominal pain that should not wait to be evaluated. Conditions like gallbladder inflammation (cholecystitis), pancreas inflammation (pancreatitis), diverticulitis, stomach ulcers, aortic dissection, bowel obstructions, and various cancers can start with abdominal pain. Unfortunately, for many abdominal conditions, there is no way to know if you may be at risk for having them except by having early screening tests that are available. There are ways to try to prevent some of the conditions listed (and other conditions) from happening, but much of the time, these conditions occur without any known risk factor(s).

TROUBLE BREATHING

It may be hard for you to imagine not seeking medical attention for trouble breathing, but it happens too often that breathing problems get explained away until the underlying cause has progressed such that it can no longer be overlooked. Sudden trouble breathing cannot be easily disregarded, but the more slowly occurring breathing problem (shortness of breath or "being winded", having trouble getting air in) can be. Common conditions like heart failure, coronary artery disease, asthma, and emphysema (COPD) can start symptomatically with a slower, progressive awareness of trying to get air in, at rest, and/or with activity.

I had a new patient with the symptom of having worsening trouble breathing for four months. He was in his 50s and had not seen a doctor in several years because his primary care doctor had retired. He was very active in sports but noticed that his ability to be active was decreasing due to having trouble breathing. He made the appointment because he could no longer ignore the symptom. Ultimately, he was found to have heart failure and diet changes and medication were instituted to treat his condition and improve his breathing problem.

Trouble breathing is often related to numerous types of heart or lung problems but can be caused by other disorders. I've had several patients in the past who came to me complaining of trouble breathing that had persisted over many months. They were found to have significant anemia from various conditions involving slow blood loss, including slow and seemingly innocuous bleeding from hemorrhoids, heavy periods and an asymptomatic bleeding stomach ulcer.

SEEING BLOOD

Seeing blood coming from your body from anywhere (other than regular menstruation) should never be ignored. Seeing blood almost always means there has been a breach of your closed circulatory system (arteries and veins) or an injury to tissue is occurring somewhere. Even something as simple as an unexplained nosebleed should at least be evaluated to see if there is something serious going on. Unexplained bleeding from any orifice (mouth, nose, eyes, ears, nipples, vaginal area, penis, rectum) and blood in stool or urine (seeing bleeding and/or with wiping) should be immediately evaluated. Bleeding does not have to be accompanied by pain to be deemed serious. I've had numerous patients that have had severe high blood pressure diagnosed for the first time after having recurrent nosebleeds but were otherwise feeling fine.

I urge you to take heed: chest pain, abdominal pain and unexplained bleeding are serious conditions that should be addressed urgently by a medical professional.

4

Make Changes Now or You May Not Have a Choice Later

*T*HIS SECTION HEADING WAS A STATEMENT THAT A PATIENT made during a visit that was scheduled to talk about making healthy food choices and to follow up on her preventive health gaps. Her exact words were *If You Don't Choose to Make Changes Now, You May Not Have a Choice Later.* She was at a point in her life where she was consistently attentive to making appropriate choices for her health today, so she would not have to "face the person" that she didn't want to be in the future. She was also reflecting on other lifestyle choices that she had made that ultimately could affect her health, like choosing to exercise or not, working on marital relations and relationships with children, and making job/career choices.

I asked her what she felt I could say to many of my other patients to encourage them to think proactively about their health as she does. She said, "Ask the question: will you be able to face/ deal with who you are and what you are later on in your life?" Ultimately, choices you make today affect what your life is and what you have to deal with tomorrow. The focus of our discussion that day was especially talking about healthy eating strategies; however, as I thought about our conversation later, I expanded on the concepts we reviewed and reworked them to share with future patients.

A good first step to making proactive life choices is to organize your eating. Daily eating plans are some of the most important decisions you can make repeatedly over the course of your life. We all have to eat and each time you eat, you have a chance to get it right or get it wrong. I have found that people don't consciously think about the decision-making that is required for eating like they do other life decisions. I encourage patients to change their relationship with food and look at eating from a paradigm of health and nourishment, instead of the vicious circle of hunger and satiety and/or emotional eating. Human beings must eat to live, so having a healthy eating strategy provides sustenance that is necessary for life today and future health tomorrow.

I remember a new patient who wanted to lose weight and control her diabetes. She was on multiple medications, including large doses of insulin, that she wanted to eliminate or at least decrease the dosage. I reviewed her history and made suggestions about how to achieve her goals with respect to making lifestyle changes and making healthier food choices. She was very motivated about changing her eating habits, and we were able to eliminate insulin and other oral medications within 4-6 weeks of our first visit. After the first visit, she sent me a patient portal message about her blood pressure and glucose (blood sugar) being too low. I told her to stop taking the insulin and eliminated one blood pressure medication. At the next visit, her blood pressure and glucose were still too low, so I eliminated the rest of her diabetes medications and eliminated a second blood pressure pill from her regimen. She was able to maintain control of her diabetes without medication (glucose readings evaluated by her checking her glucose at home every day) and only needed one blood pressure lowering medication instead of three (verified by her checking her blood pressure at home every day).

I have many patient stories like this. Changing diet can help your doctor eliminate medications that are not needed anymore. For many, the process can go very quickly. People often realize they're consuming more calories than necessary when they find themselves not hungry despite eating small amounts of healthy food more frequently. Many of my patients over the years who have changed eating habits and have subsequently lost weight and de-escalated their medication regimen tell me they feel better physically and emotionally.

In our current society, many of our social events, holidays, vacations and actually gatherings are planned around food. But you don't have to forgo the food that is consumed when you eat out, order out, or go to events because it is our everyday eating that impacts our health in the long run. You can enjoy social eating for any particular event or gathering and then go back to your regular eating when the event is over.

Supplying your body with the appropriate food is ultimately indispensable. Knowing what you are going to eat is a day-by-day and hour-by-hour continuous process. Whether you have a daily written eating plan or have a plan in your head, discerning what you are going to eat and when allows you to avoid uncontrolled eating where hunger, boredom, habit or emotion, (not health,) drives what you choose to eat in the moment. Developing the habit of organized and planned eating every day is worthwhile, as it can become a permanent and beneficial routine in your life.

Planning to eat requires consistent effort by eating regularly and avoiding skipping nutrition. Attending to proper nutrition leads to good health outcomes down the road. People who are successful with this shop with a targeted grocery list of things to buy. Then they food prep for what they are going to eat 1-3 times per week, so that the food and snacks are packaged in containers and food bags, such that they are readily available for easy meal preparation and/or are easily packable to take with them (in a portable cooler with cold packs, if needed.) This is a good practice for yourself and your family during the 7-day week. It is harder to start your work week with planned eating when your well-executed organization of planned eating has been suspended for two days over the weekend. It is also easier to not "cheat" and binge eat as much on the weekends when you have done food prepping and packing during the week. Many people do the food prepping on Sunday in preparation for the work week. For many, the additional incentive of spending less money on high fat, high calorie, high salt and expensive prepared food is an added benefit to organized eating.

When I give patients my written recommendations about food to choose and foods to avoid, I often get the response, "This is boring!" and "You don't want me to eat anything!" But when I have patients talk about what they actually eat and even have them do food diaries and write down what they eat every day, we discover what they eat is very limited and does not vary much from day to day. So many people's regular eating patterns are actually not as exciting as they think they are and often doing a food diary can reveal that you need to expand your food selections to add more variety. Patients that are successful with the routine of food prepping find that they are, in fact, not eating the same things all of the time. Food prepping for access to easy single servings allows you to not overeat as well. You actually eat less with regular, controlled eating because you are not waiting until you are "starving" to eat something. Overeating often comes with trying to satisfy extreme hunger because too much time has passed since you last supplied nutrition to your body.

You may have noticed that I have not used the word "meal" in this section. I avoid the word "meal" because many people feel overwhelmed with the idea of being able to plan "meals" every day. Instead of "meal", I use the words "food" and "nutrition" to emphasize that your body just needs nourishment, and it does not have to be a complicated or elaborate undertaking every day.

Additionally, I encourage patients to stop limiting themselves with words "breakfast", "lunch" and "dinner." From a young age, we're taught about the specific foods designated for breakfast, lunch, and dinner. As adults, we often confine our food choices to what we believe should be eaten in the morning, midday, and evening. I encourage patients to not look at choosing foods in these terms because these are man-made concepts, and the human body will use food for energy despite the category that we define and the time of day we restrict ourselves to. For example, if you like salad with chicken breast, it's okay to eat it in the morning and you don't have to eat classical breakfast food which, in this country, is often laden with fat/high in cholesterol, salt and sugar.

Whether your job requires doing service calls, working in the field and at work sites, working outside, moving from place to place in a car, working in an office setting or working at home, having healthy items already packed (and unhealthy items not in your environment, for those working from home) and available for single use eating goes a long way in preventing the need for eating "on the go." "Winging it" regularly with daily eating will almost guarantee you'll be eating foods high in salt, fat, and calories multiple times per day, week after week, month after month, and year after year. The alternative of not planning to eat and then not eating at all during the day or only eating 1-2 times a day is just as unhealthy and it will likely not get you to your health needs and goals over time. It is best to eat at regular intervals before getting hungry and not wait until hunger sets in. I recommend planning for controlled eating for nutrition's sake, instead of chasing hunger when and wherever it occurs.

Many people consider/try appetite suppressants to try to lose weight and get back on track with their health. Appetite serves as a necessary function of the human body. Appetite and the desire to eat makes you want to eat to maintain your normal biologic functions. Not having an appetite is not normal and can happen with many medical disorders and with many medication side effects. Instead of focusing on suppressing appetite, I encourage people to appreciate appetite as essential for life and to satisfy it by making healthy food selections. Supplements are meant to supplement holes in your nutrition. If you do not have holes in your nutrition then you do not need supplements.

Planning to exercise is also a worthwhile effort over the course of your life. It is a valuable habit to stay active regularly, by at least walking for 30 to 40 minutes, 3 to 5 days per week. I tell my patients to call someone on your cell phone while they are walking for exercise. If you are able to talk easily without being aware of your breathing, then you should walk faster. Wrist monitors that measure your heart rate are now readily available to give you a quick assessment of how fast your heart is beating while exercising in real-time. These monitors provide an easy way to self-monitor your exercise, so that you can maximize the impact of your exercise in the time you have planned in a target heart rate range that is safe for you.

It is also important to pay attention to your mental health and check in with a mental health professional, if needed, at regular intervals to make sure that your everyday thinking is not maladaptive or dysfunctional for you and what you are trying to accomplish in life. Often, we can have negative thoughts that impair our ability to make healthy choices, medical/health related choices and otherwise. Paying attention to healthy eating habits and regular exercise can be hindered by sadness and even mild depression, anxiety, or stress in your life. Addressing grief, anxiety and depression today can prevent you from having a future chronic medical condition that cannot be reversed.

Decisions and choices made about relationships, when and when not to conceive/father children, education, job, and careers all can ultimately affect your lifetime circumstances, ongoing state of being, peace of mind and emotional existence. Being able to consistently attend to providing good nutrition for yourself is intimately entwined with your current circumstance, which is shaped by the sum total of past choices, whether you had good options to choose from or not. Willfully evaluating life choices (as best we can) as we are making them leaves a wider range of choices and opportunities later on in life.

Even if you already have chronic medical issues, including obesity, or if you are in a life situation that you cannot change at this point, you can alter the trajectory and path of your life by making deliberate changes today.

This line of thinking brings to mind a long-time patient that had high blood pressure, diabetes and had kidney function that was getting worse as determined by his blood tests. He was not good about coming to his follow-up appointments, despite me resorting to have someone from the office call him to encourage him to come in for his appointments. One Friday morning when I was reviewing my appointments for the day, he was on the schedule, but we had not recently called him to make an appointment. The reason for the visit documented on the schedule was "abdominal pain." Of course, I had to use the visit time to review his medical issues as well, since I didn't know when I would see him again.

His blood pressure in the office was too high, but fortunately, his Hemoglobin A1C test done in the office showed that his diabetes was well controlled. He was not checking his blood pressure or glucose at home and was not eating healthy as we discussed many times before. His new abdominal pain was concerning, and he was very tender on the left side of his belly when I examined him. Because it was a Friday afternoon, I advised him to go to the ED immediately to have his symptoms evaluated. These symptoms were not something I could evaluate quick enough without blood testing and abdominal imaging testing as an outpatient. Later that evening, I was able to electronically review the records from the evaluation done in the ED. There were no abnormalities seen on the CT scan pictures of his belly, but his blood tests showed that his kidney function was getting much worse. This finding was not causing any pain, but his abdominal pain got him to come to see me which led to getting blood tests done (which I would have ordered anyway.). The results of these tests alerted us to his worsening kidney status. I had my office call him to make a follow up appointment the following week. I reviewed the evaluation in the ED with him. He said that the belly pain was gone.

To this day, I am unsure about what caused his belly pain. It has never returned, but that episode got him to come to his next two visits. He told me that finding out about his worsening kidney function "scared me" and since that visit, he has changed his eating habits and has intentionally lost weight. He has been checking his blood pressure and glucose at home as instructed and his blood pressure is much better. Having good control of blood pressure and diabetes can prevent and at least delay the progression of kidney disease. Unfortunately, his kidney function had progressed to a stage where I felt the need to refer him to a kidney specialist (a nephrologist). His kidney function will likely not improve at this point, but we can at least continue to work together to prevent it from progressing to avoid end-stage kidney disease and dialysis. His experience is an example of how a medical condition can worsen to a point where choices become increasingly limited.

My patient's advice to me about making proactive health choices was to give me her perspective on how to help me encourage people to make purposeful choices today before the choice is no longer an option. The more time you let pass without making healthy choices, the more you lose the ability to choose PREVENTION of circumstances and conditions instead of TREATMENT of conditions, that could lead to a healthier future lifestyle. Choosing PREVENTION is always better than choosing TREATMENT options.

5

Health is Not About Ordering Tests

*T*HE MOST IMPORTANT THING YOU CAN DO TO PREVENT illness and disease is to pay attention to what you eat and how much cardio exercise you incorporate into your daily routine. Instead, many patients focus on what tests are being ordered by their doctor and/or asking the doctor to order tests. Invariably, at least 1-2 times per week in a new patient and/or preventive health visit, I have a patient say that they want me to "order everything" or say, "I want annual routine tests." Maintaining health and preventing illness is not just about doing testing. In fact, the only routine blood testing that is currently recommended for adults is at least a blood glucose test for diabetes screening every 3 years and checking cholesterol at least every 5 years. (United States Preventive Health Task Force-USPHTF :https://www.uspreventiveservicestaskforce.org/uspstf/ and ABIM Choose Wisely https://www.choosingwisely.org/our-mission/history/)

Any other blood testing should be ordered based on the patient's individual risk factors, medical conditions, or family history. The only truly annual preventive health recommendations left anymore for all adults are an Influenza vaccine every fall and a mammogram for women every year starting at age 40.

There is no science behind doing the "annual physical" or getting "routine" tests every year and there never was. I'm sure this is a surprise to you, but it's true. There are many things that we used to do by nothing other than habit and convention in medicine and much of that has been done away with. The focus of medical practice has been redirected over the last 20 years to use scientific evidence, as best we can, to make medical decisions that have been shown to have benefits and to stop doing things that will not be useful and/or may cause harm. Medical societies and collaborations with physicians and patients have concentrated on following updated practice guidelines that emphasize only ordering testing that is beneficial vs. unnecessary testing.

I recommend reviewing preventive health gaps at every visit with your primary care physician, such that it is not just an "annual" topic. Many physician practices have patient portals that display preventive health recommendations for you so you can keep up with what testing you are due for and when. I still do recommend a preventive health or wellness visit to be at least, if nothing else, the one visit in the year to review eating habits, exercise habits and preventive health guidelines, the patient's overall health, health goals, and priorities to target for the upcoming year. This is also a good time to review symptoms and chronic medical conditions in order to set up and/or reinforce a plan for ordering lab tests and other testing for monitoring and management of chronic conditions.

Here are the preventive health recommendations that I recommend by age group (based on United States Preventive Services Task Force USPSTF guidelines). There are some similarities and also some differences as the age group progresses.

These preventive health guidelines were up to date at the time of publishing. Please check with a qualified and licensed physician for the most up to date preventive health recommendations that apply to, as these recommendations change as medical knowledge changes regarding disease screening techniques and disease risk.

PREVENTIVE ITEM	FEMALE LESS THAN 30	FEMALE AGE 30-49	MALE AGE LESS THAN 50	FEMALE AGE 50 AND ABOVE	MALE AGE 50 AND ABOVE
Health Maintenance Examination (HME) every year					
Breast exam by your doctor once a year. Annual mammogram starting at age 40. I recommend that you do your self-breast exam once a month (7-10 days after your period, if you still have periods).					
PAP test at least every 3 years from age 21-30 and a PAP and HPV test at least every 5 years from age 30-65. If your PAP or HPV test is abnormal, your cervical cancer screening schedule will change depending upon the abnormality found.					

PREVENTIVE ITEM	FEMALE LESS THAN 30	FEMALE AGE 30-49	MALE AGE LESS THAN 50	FEMALE AGE 50 AND ABOVE	MALE AGE 50 AND ABOVE
Vaccination with HPV (human papillomavirus) vaccine is recommended for all girls/boys and women/men, starting at age 11 until at least age 26. A discussion about HPV vaccination up to age 45 should be based on an individual's risk factors.	▓	▓	▓	▓	▓
Vaccination against tetanus includes a tetanus-diphtheria vaccination booster (Td) every 10 years with a tetanus-diphtheria-pertussis/whooping cough vaccination (Tdap) on one occasion during adulthood.	▓	▓	▓	▓	▓
Influenza vaccine is offered every Fall starting in October.	▓	▓	▓	▓	▓
Pneumococcal vaccination (vaccination against the pneumococcus bacteria that causes severe pneumonias) is recommended starting at age 65. Prevnar 20, Prevnar 13 and Pneumovax are commonly used names of this type of vaccination. It is also recommended in all diabetics (and for people with other chronic diseases and smokers) at least once prior to age 65.	▓	▓	▓	▓	▓
A Shingles vaccine (Shingrix) is recommended starting at age 50.				▓	▓
Screening for diabetes at least every 3 years	▓	▓	▓	▓	▓
Cholesterol screening at least every 5 years	▓	▓	▓	▓	▓

PREVENTIVE ITEM	FEMALE LESS THAN 30	FEMALE AGE 30-49	MALE AGE LESS THAN 50	FEMALE AGE 50 AND ABOVE	MALE AGE 50 AND ABOVE
HIV test at least once in all adults and other sexually diseases, such as Hepatitis B, Hepatitis C and syphilis infections. I routinely screen for Chlamydia and gonorrhea depending on risk and sexual behavior.	■	■	■	■	■
Complete eye exam at least once a year to screen for glaucoma and more often depending on medical conditions.	■	■	■	■	■
Colon cancer screening with a colonoscopy (a test to look inside the colon to find polyps that can turn into colon cancer) is recommended starting at least by age 45.		■	■	■	■
A bone density test at least starting at age 65 to screen for osteoporosis				■	
Annual lung cancer screening: 50 to 80 years of age, a family history of lung cancer, smoking history at least 20 pack years or more AND current smokers or former smokers who quit smoking within the past 15 years.				■	■
Have a discussion with your doctor about whether prostate cancer screening with a digital rectal exam (DRE) and prostate blood test (PSA) is appropriate for you.			■		■
Ultrasound of the abdominal aorta is recommended for men over 50 who have EVER SMOKED to look for an aneurysm.					■

WOMEN LESS THAN 30

I recommend a Health Maintenance Examination (HME) and/ or Well Woman Exam every year to update your health history, including illnesses, medications, allergies, review any new or old symptoms and changes in your sexual habits and overall function. I perform an exam (a pelvic exam is not recommended every year anymore), including checking blood pressure and pulse and performing other evaluations, as indicated by your age, risks and health issues.

I recommend that I examine your breasts once a year. I recommend an annual mammogram starting at age 40. I recommend that you do your self-breast exam once a month (7-10 days after your period, if you still have periods).

Current cervical cancer screening guidelines include a PAP test at least every 3 years from age 21-30 and a PAP and HPV test at least every 5 years from age 30-65. (https://www.us-preventiveservicestaskforce.org/uspstf/recommendation/ cervical-cancer-screening) If your PAP or HPV test is abnormal, your cervical cancer screening schedule will change depending upon the abnormality found. I routinely screen for Chlamydia and gonorrhea depending on your risks and sexual history.

Vaccination with HPV (human papillomavirus) vaccine is recommended for all girls/boys and women/men, starting at age 11 until at least age 26. A discussion about HPV vaccination up to age 45 should be based on an individual's risk factors. HPV is a common sexually transmitted virus in the United States and affects over 50% of sexually active men and women at some point in their lives. (https://www.cdc.gov/mmwr/volumes/68/wr/ mm6832a3.htm) It causes genital and anal warts and cervical and anal cancer. Vaccination may help prevent these problems. This vaccine protects against the 4 strains that cause 75-90% of cervical and anal cancers. Since few women have been exposed to all 4 strains, the vaccine is even important for women with a past history of HPV.

Vaccination against tetanus includes a tetanus-diphtheria vaccination booster (Td) every 10 years with a tetanus-diphtheria-pertussis/whooping cough vaccination (Tdap) on one occasion during adulthood.

The influenza vaccine is offered every Fall starting in October. It is strongly recommended for adults with chronic health issues like diabetes, heart disease, lung disease, liver disease, HIV infection and other chronic medical conditions.

Pneumococcal vaccination (vaccination against the pneumococcus bacteria that causes severe pneumonias) is recommended starting at age 65. Prevnar 20, Prevnar 13 and Pneumovax are commonly used names of this type of vaccination. It is also recommended for all diabetics (and for people with other chronic diseases and smokers) at least once prior to age 65. (https://www.cdc.gov/vaccines/hcp/acip-recs/vacc-specific/pneumo.html)

Other vaccination recommendations depend on your risks, health history and travel plans.

The only two routine blood tests that are recommended are:

- Screening for diabetes by at least checking a blood sugar (blood glucose) every three years.
- Screening for high cholesterol at least every 5 years and more frequently depending on the results and your history.
- Any other testing that I may recommend will depend on any symptoms you have or your medical history.

I recommend checking for HIV at least once in all adults and other sexually diseases, such as Hepatitis B, Hepatitis C and syphilis infections. These are all sexually transmitted diseases that you can have for many years and not have any symptoms. Checking for Hepatitis C is now recommended at least for all adults born between 1945 and 1965. In 2020, this guideline was updated to include screening all persons aged 18-79. (https://www.uspreventiveservicestaskforce.org/uspstf/recommendation/hepatitis-c-screening)

I recommend a complete eye exam at least once a year to screen for glaucoma and more often depending on your history.

WOMEN AGED 30 – 49

I recommend a Health Maintenance Examination (HME) and/or Well Woman Exam to update your health history, including illnesses, medications, allergies, review any new or old symptoms and changes in your sexual habits and overall function. I perform an exam (a pelvic exam is not recommended every year anymore), including checking blood pressure and pulse and performing other evaluations, as indicated by your age, risks and health issues.

I recommend that I examine your breasts once a year. I recommend an annual mammogram starting at age 40. I recommend that you do your self-breast exam once a month (7-10 days after your period, if you still have periods).

There are new cervical cancer screening guidelines that went into effect in 2013:

Current cervical cancer screening guidelines include a PAP test at least every 3 years from age 21-30 and a PAP and HPV test every 5 years from age 30-65. If your PAP or HPV test is abnormal, your cervical cancer screening schedule will change depending upon the abnormality found. I routinely screen for Chlamydia and gonorrhea depending on your risks and sexual history.

A discussion about HPV vaccination up to age 45 should be based on an individual's risk factors. HPV is a common sexually transmitted virus in the United States and affects over 50% of sexually active men and women at some point in their lives. It causes genital and anal warts and cervical and anal cancer. Vaccination may help prevent these problems. This vaccine protects against the 4 strains that cause 75-90% of cervical and anal cancers. Since few women have been exposed to all 4 strains, the vaccine is even important for women with a past history of HPV.

Vaccination against tetanus includes a tetanus-diphtheria vaccination booster (Td) every 10 years with a tetanus-diphtheria-pertussis/whooping cough vaccination (Tdap) on one occasion during adulthood.

The influenza vaccine is offered every Fall starting in October. It is strongly recommended for adults with chronic health issues like diabetes, heart disease, lung disease, liver disease, HIV infection and other chronic medical conditions.

Pneumococcal vaccination (vaccination against the pneumococcus bacteria that causes severe pneumonias) is recommended starting at age 65. Prevnar 20, Prevnar 13 and Pneumovax are commonly used names of this type of vaccination. It is also recommended in all diabetics (and for people with other chronic diseases and smokers) at least once prior to age 65.

Other vaccination recommendations depend on your risks, health history and travel plans.

Colon cancer screening by doing a colonoscopy (a test to look inside the colon to find polyps that can turn into colon cancer) is recommended starting at least by age 45 (and earlier depending on your risk) and at least every 10 years after that until at least age 75. Finding certain types of polyps in the colon will require more frequent repeat testing depending on the findings in the colon. There are other options for colon cancer screening that are less effective that you should discuss with your doctor. (https://www.uspreventiveservicestaskforce.org/uspstf/recommendation/colorectal-cancer-screening)

The only two routine blood tests that are recommended are:

- Screening for diabetes by at least checking a blood sugar (blood glucose) every three years.
- Screening for high cholesterol at least every 5 years and more frequently depending on the results and your history.
- Any other testing that I may recommend will depend on any symptoms you have or your medical history.

I recommend checking for HIV at least once in all adults and other sexually diseases, such as Hepatitis B, Hepatitis C and syphilis infections. These are all sexually transmitted diseases that you can have for many years and not have any symptoms. Checking for Hepatitis C is now recommended at least for all adults born between 1945 and 1965. In 2020, this guideline was updated to include screening all persons aged 18-79.

I recommend a complete eye exam at least once to screen for glaucoma and more often depending on your history.

WOMEN AGED 50 AND OLDER

I recommend a Health Maintenance Examination (HME) and/or Well Woman Exam to update your health history, including illnesses, medications, allergies, review any new or old symptoms and changes in your sexual habits and overall function. I perform an exam (a pelvic exam is not recommended every year anymore), including checking blood pressure and pulse and performing other evaluations, as indicated by your age, risks and health issues. If you have Medicare and are 65 years old and above, an Annual Wellness Visit is your covered benefit for your annual preventive health visit.

I recommend that I examine your breasts once a year. I recommend an annual mammogram starting at age 40. I recommend that you do your self-breast exam once a month (7-10 days after your period, if you still have periods).

There are updated cervical cancer screening guidelines that went into effect in 2013:

Current cervical cancer screening guidelines include a PAP and HPV test every 5 years age 30-65. If your PAP or HPV test is abnormal, your cervical cancer screening schedule will change depending upon the abnormality found. I routinely screen for Chlamydia and gonorrhea depending on your risks and sexual history.

Vaccination against tetanus includes a tetanus-diphtheria vaccination booster (Td) every 10 years with a tetanus-diphtheria-pertussis/whooping cough vaccination (Tdap) on one occasion during adulthood.

The influenza vaccine is offered every Fall starting in October. It is strongly recommended for adults with chronic health issues like diabetes, heart disease, lung disease, liver disease, HIV infection, and other chronic medical conditions.

A Shingles vaccine (Shingrix) is recommended starting at age 50. It is a two-injection series that you should get at your local retail pharmacy or in your doctor's office. (https://www.cdc.gov/vaccines/hcp/acip-recs/vacc-specific/shingles.html)

Pneumococcal vaccination (vaccination against the pneumococcus bacteria that causes severe pneumonias) is recommended starting at age 65. Prevnar 20, Prevnar 13 and Pneumovax are commonly used names of this type of vaccination. It is also recommended in all diabetics (and for people with other chronic diseases and smokers) at least once prior to age 65.

Other vaccination recommendations depend on your risks, health history and travel plans.

A bone density test should be done at least starting at age 65 to screen for osteoporosis. I make other individual recommendations about osteoporosis screening and taking calcium and Vitamin D supplements depending on age, history and past bone density findings. (https://www.uspreventiveservicestaskforce.org/uspstf/recommendation/osteoporosis-screening)

Colon cancer screening by doing a colonoscopy (a test to look inside the colon to find polyps that can turn into colon cancer) is recommended starting at least by age 45 (and earlier depending on your risk) and at least every 10 years after that until at least age 75. Finding certain types of polyps in the colon will require more frequent repeat testing depending on the findings in the colon. There are other options for colon cancer screening that are less effective that you should discuss with your doctor.

Patients who meet the following screening criteria may be at high risk for lung cancer and may benefit from annual lung cancer screening:

- 50 to 80 years of age
- A family history of lung cancer

- Smoking history at least 20 pack years (This is the number of years you smoked multiplied by the number of packs of cigarettes per day. For example, someone who smoked 2 packs per day for 15 years [2 × 15 = 30] has 30 pack-years of smoking. A person who smoked 1 pack per day for 30 years [1 × 30 = 30] also has 30 pack-years of smoking) or more AND current smokers or former smokers who quit smoking within the past 15 years. (https://www.cancer.org/cancer/lung-cancer/detection-diagnosis-staging/detection.html)

The only two routine blood tests that are recommended (any other testing that I may recommend will depend on any symptoms you have or your medical history) are:

- Screening for diabetes by at least checking a blood sugar (blood glucose) every three years.
- Screening for high cholesterol at least every 5 years and more frequently depending on the results and your history.
- Any other testing that I may recommend will depend on any symptoms you have or your medical history.

I recommend checking for HIV at least once in all adults and other sexually diseases, such as Hepatitis B, Hepatitis C and syphilis infections. These are all sexually transmitted diseases that you can have for many years without experiencing any symptoms. Checking for Hepatitis C is now recommended at least for all adults born between 1945 and 1965. In 2020, this guideline was updated to include screening all persons, age 18-79.

I recommend a complete eye exam at least once to screen for glaucoma and more often depending on your history.

MEN LESS THAN AGE 50

I recommend a Health Maintenance Examination (HME) or wellness visit at least every 1-3 years to update your health history, including illnesses, medications, allergies, review any new or old symptoms and changes in your sexual habits and overall function. I perform an exam, including checking blood pressure and pulse and perform other evaluations as indicated by your age, risks and health issues.

Vaccination against tetanus includes a tetanus-diphtheria vaccination booster (Td) every 10 years with a tetanus-diphtheria-pertussis/whooping cough vaccination (Tdap) on one occasion during adulthood.

The influenza vaccine is offered every Fall starting in October. It is strongly recommended for adults with chronic health issues like diabetes, heart disease, lung disease, liver disease, HIV infection, and other chronic medical conditions.

Other vaccination recommendations depend on your risks, health history and travel plans.

Vaccination with HPV (human papillomavirus) vaccine is recommended for all girls/boys and women/men, starting at age 11 until at least age 26. A discussion about HPV vaccination up to age 45 should be based on an individual's risk factors. HPV is a common sexually transmitted virus in the United States and affects over 50% of sexually active men and women at some point in their lives. It causes genital and anal warts and cervical and anal cancer. Vaccination may help prevent these problems for you or your partner. This vaccine protects against the 4 strains that cause 75-90% of cervical and anal cancers.

Pneumococcal vaccination (vaccination against the pneumococcus bacteria that causes severe pneumonias) is recommended starting at age 65. Prevnar 20, Prevnar 13 and Pneumovax are commonly used names of this type of vaccination. It is also recommended for all diabetics (and for people with other chronic diseases and smokers) at least once prior to age 65.

Colon cancer screening by doing a colonoscopy (a test to look inside the colon to find polyps that can turn into colon cancer) is recommended starting at least by age 45 (and earlier depending on your risk) and at least every 10 years after that until at least age 75. Finding certain types of polyps in the colon will require more frequent repeat testing depending on the findings in the colon. There are other options for colon cancer screening that are less effective that you should discuss with your doctor.

You should have a discussion with your doctor about whether prostate cancer screening with a digital rectal exam (DRE) and prostate blood test (PSA) is appropriate for you. I discuss prostate cancer screening in more detail in the next section. (https://www.cancer.org/cancer/prostate-cancer/detection-diagnosis-staging/acs-recommendations.html)

The only two routine blood tests that are recommended (any other testing that I may recommend will depend on any symptoms you have or your medical history) are:

- Screening for diabetes by at least checking a blood sugar (blood glucose) every three years.
- Screening for high cholesterol at least every 5 years and more frequently depending on the results and your history.

- Any other testing that I may recommend will depend on any symptoms you have or your medical history.

I recommend checking for HIV at least once in all adults and other sexually diseases, such as Hepatitis B, Hepatitis C and syphilis infections. These are all sexually transmitted diseases that you can have for many years and not have any symptoms. Checking for Hepatitis C is now recommended at least for all adults born between 1945 and 1965. In 2020, this guideline was updated to include screening all persons aged 18-79.

I recommend a complete eye exam at least once to screen for glaucoma and more often depending on your history.

MEN AGED 50 AND OLDER

I recommend a Health Maintenance Examination (HME) every year to update your health history, including illnesses, medications, allergies, review any new or old symptoms and changes in your sexual habits and overall function. I perform an exam, including checking blood pressure and pulse and perform other evaluations as indicated by your age, risks and health issues. If you have Medicare, an Annual Wellness Visit is your covered benefit for your annual preventive health visit.

Vaccination against tetanus includes a tetanus-diphtheria vaccination booster (Td) every 10 years with a tetanus-diphtheria-pertussis/whooping cough vaccination (Tdap) on one occasion during adulthood.

The influenza vaccine is offered every Fall starting in October. It is strongly recommended for adults with chronic health issues like diabetes, heart disease, lung disease, liver disease, HIV infection, and other chronic medical conditions.

A Shingles vaccine (Shingrix) is recommended starting at age 50. It is a two-injection series that you should get at your local retail pharmacy or in your doctor's office.

Pneumococcal vaccination (vaccination against the pneumococcus bacteria that causes severe pneumonias) is recommended starting at age 65. Prevnar 13 and Pneumovax are commonly used names of this type of vaccination. It is also recommended for all diabetics (and for people with other chronic diseases and smokers) at least once prior to age 65.

Other vaccination recommendations depend on your risks, health history and travel plans.

Colon cancer screening by doing a colonoscopy (a test to look inside the colon to find polyps that can turn into colon cancer) is recommended starting at least by age 45 (and earlier depending on your risk) and at least every 10 years after that until at least age 75. Finding certain types of polyps in the colon will require more frequent repeat testing depending on the findings in the colon. There are other options for colon cancer screening that are less effective that you should discuss with your doctor.

You should have a discussion with your doctor about whether prostate cancer screening with a digital rectal exam (DRE) and prostate blood test (PSA) is appropriate for you. (https://www.uspreventiveservicestaskforce.org/uspstf/recommendation/prostate-cancer-screening).

THE PROSTATE CANCER SCREENING CONUNDRUM

For some men, prostate cancer screening offers a chance to catch aggressive cancers before it is too late. Therefore, the PSA screening test can be a life saver. At the same time, prostate cancer screening can lead to both benefits and harms. PSA screening subjects thousands of men every year to biopsies and other medical procedures that carry the risk of bleeding and infection and cause unnecessary anxiety. Furthermore, screening leads to treatment of a lot of cancers that are not life threatening. In addition, the treatments can cause impotence and incontinence and seriously erode a man's quality of life.

The issues surrounding PSA testing are conflicting because although many men are diagnosed with prostate cancer, most of them do not die from their cancer. Prostate cancer often progresses so slowly that many men die from other causes before they even develop symptoms of the disease.

Ask yourself the following questions when deciding whether or not to be screened for prostate cancer:

- Am I at high risk for prostate cancer?
- Do I want to know if I have prostate cancer?
- How do I feel about the possibility of getting a "false positive" result?
- Am I willing to have a prostate biopsy to check for cancer?
- Would I want to be treated if I learned I had prostate cancer?
- How do I feel about the risks of being treated for prostate cancer?
- How would I feel about getting a serious (or even deadly) form of prostate cancer if I had decided not to get screened?

https://www.uptodate.com/contents/prostate-cancer-screening-beyond-the-basics?topicRef=7567&source=see_link
(Table 1)

An ultrasound of your abdominal aorta is recommended for men over 50 who have EVER SMOKED to look for an aneurysm. Men who smoke are at higher risk of having aneurysms of the aorta. Aneurysms can break open and bleed and cause serious problems.

Patients who meet the following screening criteria may be at high risk for lung cancer and may benefit from annual lung cancer screening:

- 50 to 80 years of age
- A family history of lung cancer
- Smoking history at least 20 pack years (This is the number of years you smoked multiplied by the number of packs of cigarettes per day. For example, someone who smoked 2 packs per day for 15 years $[2 \times 15 = 30]$ has 30 pack-years of smoking. A person who smoked 1 pack per day for 30 years $[1 \times 30 = 30]$ also has 30 pack-years of smoking) or more AND current smokers or former smokers who quit smoking within the past 15 years.

The only two routine blood tests that are recommended (any other testing that I may recommend will depend on any symptoms you have or your medical history) are:

- Screening for diabetes by at least checking a blood sugar (blood glucose) every three years.
- Screening for high cholesterol at least every 5 years and more frequently depending on the results and your history.
- Any other testing that I may recommend will depend on any symptoms you have or your medical history.

I recommend checking for HIV at least once in all adults and other sexually diseases, such as Hepatitis B, Hepatitis C and syphilis infections. These are all sexually transmitted diseases that you can have for many years and not have any symptoms. Checking for Hepatitis C is now recommended at least for all adults born between 1945 and 1965. In 2020, this guideline was updated to include screening all persons aged 18-79.

I recommend a complete eye exam at least once to screen for glaucoma and more often depending on your history.

6

The Patient Is Not Always Right

*T*HIS CHAPTER CAME ABOUT DUE TO THE MANY TIMES patients have asked for a medication or treatment that I thought was not safe or inappropriate. I do remember a patient telling me once that, "The patient is always right." I responded to him that the patient *is not always right* and then I explained to him the medical basis for my assertion and why I declined to order what he was asking for. I wish the patient was always right. It would make things so much easier.

When I thought about the conversation later, what I should have said is that it's not about being "right" at all. What is more important is that when doing a medical evaluation, the plan for the evaluation should proceed as correctly, safely, and logically as possible following current guidelines and best scientific evidence. When I have a patient ask for a treatment, test, or medication, I always ask where they heard about it and what concerns they have that caused them to make their request. This helps me get to the basis of what the patient is asking for. Often, what patients request may not be suitable for their needs, but addressing their underlying concerns is essential. It's not about right or wrong, but about ensuring the patient receives the appropriate assessment and evaluation, if necessary.

As a physician, it's my task to reconcile the patient's anxieties with what is really concerning them. Patients often make decisions based on feeling and emotion. Their concerns and expectations must be clarified so that the appropriate decision about testing can be made. This takes time, but it's worth it to avoid patient misunderstanding, confusion, and feeling that concerns are not being addressed. It is also an opportunity to find out what the patient's health concerns really are. Frequently, once the patient's particular concerns are addressed, we conclude that no testing needs to be done at all.

I can remember a patient that made an appointment with me to request a prescription for a medication, Propranolol, that a friend of hers was taking for (tremors) shaking. The patient didn't know anything about her friend's medical history or why she was taking the medication. Upon further questioning, my patient revealed that she began experiencing shaking of her head six months before the visit, and the shaking in her hands started two months prior to the visit. She said she never mentioned it to me during our initial visit previously because it was so mild, such that she only *felt* the shaking more than she or anyone else could *see* the shaking. The shaking was still mild, but it was present enough that it was starting to affect her handwriting and opening jars. I asked about other symptoms, and she mentioned she had started losing weight without intentionally trying to do so, and she had not made any changes to her eating or exercise routines. I told her that prescribing the requested medication would not be appropriate until we evaluated the cause of her symptoms. She was disappointed that she left the visit without the prescription, but she agreed to get the blood tests done that I ordered.

The outcome of the evaluation is that she had an overactive thyroid function (hyperthyroidism) and treatment of her hyperthyroidism resolved her shaking. Just taking the medication she requested without doing the evaluation may have resolved her shaking, but would have left her hyperthyroidism undiagnosed and untreated. This would have had serious implications for her health very soon.

7

Advice for the Decades

I N MY PRACTICE, I BEGIN TAKING CARE OF PATIENTS FROM the age of eighteen all the way into their senior years. There is a typical pattern of experiences that many people have over the course of their life that impacts the discussions I have with patients about health, illness, wellness, and well-being.

These life issues build upon the previous decade(s) and/or past history. Based on these patterns I have observed by taking care of patients longitudinally, these are general recommendations that I have for people to consider when making decisions as you progress through your life journey.

AGE 18 TO 30

- Avoid unplanned pregnancy and unplanned fathering of children unless you are ready to fully commit to nurturing, raising, supporting, and caring for another individual. For pregnancy prevention, condoms are your first line of defense for STD's and controlling when you get pregnant or father children. In addition, there are hormonal and non-hormonal forms of birth control including pills, injections, implants, IUDs, and permanent forms of contraception like tubal ligation for women and vasectomy for men. You should discuss with your primary care physician or OB/GYN about which method is best for you. Men and women should be open with sexual partners about their feelings regarding becoming a parent and their current desire to get pregnant, not get pregnant, father children or not father children.

- Prevent sexually transmitted infections (STI's) by consistently using condoms and developing habits for consistently (every time) preventing sexually transmitted disease by limiting sexual partners and being direct with asking questions of sexual partners about their sexual practices. I recommend that sexual partners be tested for STI's and results be shared between you and your sexual partners. I often must educate patients in this age group with talking points about getting this kind of information from potential sexual partners and about being comfortable asking these questions. You should talk to your doctor about what questions you should be asking sexual partners and about how to share information about yourself to potential sexual partners. I recommend you do not have sex if you do not get satisfactory answers to your questions or if the person is not willing to get STI's testing with you before becoming sexually intimate. Have the conversation in a neutral environment and emphasize in a caring manner that you want to protect yourself and your partner from a sexually transmitted infection going forward.

TALKING POINTS TO DISCUSS SEXUAL HISTORY WITH A POTENTIAL OR CURRENT PARTNER:

- Do you use latex (not sheepskin—HIV can penetrate sheepskin condoms) condoms/barrier method (female condom, dental dam) EVERY TIME you have sex with someone else to protect yourself from STI's with oral, vaginal or anal sex?
- Have you ever been tested for or diagnosed with an STI? Which infection? Did you complete the entire treatment that was prescribed or are you currently taking the recommended medication/treatment as prescribed?
- When was the last time that you were checked for HIV? Hepatitis B? Hepatitis C? Syphilis? Chlamydia? Gonorrhea?
- Do you take or have you taken pills in the past to prevent HIV or PrEP (PrEP or pre-exposure prophylaxis) is prescription medication designed to prevent HIV infection. It can be prescribed to HIV-negative people who have sex with HIV-positive individuals or those at high risk of infection.) (https://www.healthgrades. com/right-care/sexual-health/9-questions-to-ask-about-your-partners-sexual-history) and (https://www. plannedparenthood.org/learn/stds-hiv-safer-sex/ get-tested/how-do-i-talk-my-partner-about-std-testing)
- Getting pregnant and fathering children is always better and less high risk the healthier you are. Keeping an appropriate weight, eating healthy, getting regular exercise, avoiding smoking and substance use, including marijuana and alcohol improves the chances of getting pregnant

or fathering children and having a healthy pregnancy and healthy child. Pre-natal planning and consultation with an OB/GYN can maximize your ability to have healthy pregnancy outcomes.

- Avoid developing unhealthy habits like smoking, increased alcohol use and drug use that alters your mental status. I include marijuana for recreational use in this recommendation. I don't see a lot of patients that start tobacco smoking habits if they have not started by age 25, but I often see patients develop dysfunctional alcohol use habits in their 30s and 40s. Alcohol and drug use, including marijuana use, can alter your mental status in life at crucial points where important choices need to be made with a clear mind. As a physician, I feel that in the long term, too much alcohol intake is more harmful than marijuana use, but marijuana use on a regular basis is not without consequences. Regular marijuana use can impair the ability to form memories, which is not a small matter and may not be reversible. Substances that are mind altering (such as cocaine, heroin, crystal meth, LSD and other hallucinogenic drugs) and even abuse of prescription drugs that alter mental status can lead to all types of problems in life. Dependence and addiction negatively affect relationships, causing poor job performance, job loss, your ability to provide for yourself and your family and maintaining independence.

- Invest as much as you can in education and skill training during your 20s. Education can take all types of forms and does not only mean a formal college or university education. Getting some type of training is very useful in developing marketable skills that somebody will pay you for, whether you are going to work for someone else or work for yourself. Being able to provide for yourself and your family goes a long way to alleviating future stress and keeping doors open for yourself and keeping choices available for yourself in the future. Education and training decisions that you make in your 20s can affect your health for years to come.

- Often people choose life partners and spouses in their 20s before knowing who they really are. It is hard to choose a partner for yourself when you do not know yourself. Unfortunately, when a life partner is chosen in the 20s, the person who you are aware of is often different than the person that you really are. Try to pay attention to what type of person you are developing into. Over the course of my career, I have heard many patients lament (and proclaim) life partner choices they made in their 20s are still negatively impacting them today.

- Start developing regular, healthy eating habits and getting regular exercise. The health that you can develop in your 20s goes a long way to determining what your health will be like for the rest of your life. This is a time in your life where you should start getting regular preventive health visits to know if your blood pressure, cholesterol or glucose (blood sugar) is elevated. I meet many patients in this age group that have already started to have issues with pre-diabetes, diabetes, elevated blood pressure, obesity and high cholesterol.

- Talk to your parents and grandparents and cousins about their medical issues and their parents' medical conditions before they get too old to remember or start to pass away. Write down your family history of medical illnesses and share this information with your siblings so that your family history can be given to your doctors. Knowledge of family history helps your doctor know what to look out for as you get older.

- Get all of your pediatric records either from your pediatrician or from your parents. Usually, it is your mother who will have this information hidden away somewhere in her house. You are an adult now and it is time for you to be the guardian of these records instead of your mother. And your pediatrician does not need them anymore. This is important regardless of your age. Many symptoms, testing and illnesses occurring in childhood have implications well into adulthood.

- This is often a time in adults where psychotic and mood disorders like schizophrenia, bipolar disorder, anxiety, and depression start. ADHD becomes difficult to manage and compensate for when work, school and/or life responsibilities start to increase. Unfortunately, no one has control over these conditions, but this is the decade in life where the symptoms of these conditions can begin, if they have not already started in childhood or in adolescence. Others may tell you that they have noticed changes in your behavior. If you notice changes in your thinking or how you process information, I recommend discussing your feelings with your doctor to determine if further evaluation is necessary. There are good treatments (medication and non-medication therapy) that are currently available to help, such that a mental health condition does not have to incapacitate your life.

- This is the age group where what you have envisioned for your life starts to move away from the reality of how your life is going. This can cause lots of worry and anxiety as you start to have to accept what you may have planned for your life is not what your life is going to be. Despite this, this can also be an exciting time in life where you may find your goals have adjusted to something greater than what you did not think of before. At this age group, I often have to encourage people to let go of worrying about things and people that they cannot change. This is the time in life where people become more aware of what is going on in the global environment and how much of what is going on in the world is unpleasant and frightening. I encourage people to re-focus on their life and what they can contribute to their own personal environment can bring meaning and gratification to them going forward.

AGE 31–40

- This is the time of your life when you really get to know your body and what feels normal and what does not. You are better able to know what abnormal symptoms are for you and when to seek medical attention to have them addressed.
- This is also a time that many people go back to school, are raising children, advancing careers, and are getting settled into a job or vocation. This is often a good time in life to enjoy health-wise, before chronic medical issues start to happen, which can encumber enjoyment in life. It is also a time where managing chronic medical issues starts to be more challenging if they were not managed in the previous decade of your life.

- As I've noted previously, now is the time to be very focused about maintaining healthy eating habits and getting regular exercise. Solidifying good eating and exercise habits at this time of life will go a long way to form the foundation of your health to support disease prevention in the future.

- This is also the time to plan pregnancies and/or fathering children. Also, this is the time to consider freezing your eggs or sperm if you are planning to delay childbearing and fathering children.

- This is a time in life where people start working on saving money for the future and/or planning and implementing a strategy to invest (retirement savings through employers, buying real estate, buying your first home, starting a business, etc.). People also buy life, long term care, and disability insurance and implement estate planning at this time with the intention of passing on wealth and assets to family in the event that death occurs. It can be a source of anxiety to begin to think about your own mortality. The sooner this can be started, the better you can feel about finances as you get older. People start to have more anxiety and stress about finances in the future as they get older.

- This is a good time to start talking to family members about your wishes in the event that you become so ill that you cannot make medical decisions for yourself (Living Will and Advanced Directives). People in their 20-40's often die of sudden accidents, homicide and suicide, where there is no advance time for family to discuss your wishes with you. Making your wishes known to your health care designee and having it written down goes a long way to make sure that your wishes are carried out and the person that you have designated can carry out your wishes. (See section on Advanced Directives for details.)

- This is also the time of life where the onset of symptoms of chronic medical conditions begins to occur. These are conditions that you have no control over, cannot prevent, screen for or diagnose early. This is the time when disorders like lupus, other underlying inflammatory conditions, multiple sclerosis, inflammatory bowel disease and other inflammatory or degenerative conditions begin. Thyroid disorders often start at this time, if they have not started already. Chronic diseases you cannot see and don't have symptoms of yet, also begin to occur. Conditions like diabetes and conditions that are a result of artery disease/blockage of arteries (heart disease, strokes, kidney disease, peripheral vascular disease {blocked arteries in the neck, legs large arteries in the chest and abdomen}) start slowly at this time. There are no symptoms of this disease progression until 15-20 years from now, but this is the time to be mindful of your diet and exercise. If you are a smoker, quitting can prevent or at least delay the onset and/or decrease the severity of these conditions if they occur later in life.

- Mental health conditions that have not been adequately or consistently addressed earlier in life frequently begin to be difficult to manage and this regularly comes to the attention of the primary care physician. People often start discussing this with their primary physician to get help with referrals to a mental health provider and advice on management options. The most common conditions are anxiety and depression which may have started earlier in life or sometimes life circumstances or life issues bring the symptoms to the forefront. Sometimes people start to have more difficulty coping with the increasing complexities in life. Often people have tried to manage symptoms on their own but start to have problems with doing so.

• This is a good time in life to be intentional about developing good sleep habits.

AGE 41–50

• This age bracket begins the annual screening processes. For women, it's the start of getting annual mammograms. For both women and men, colon cancer screening is starting at age 45. This is a good time to make sure you have a preventive health visit and/or wellness visit with your primary care physician at least once a year to screen for the onset of high blood pressure, high cholesterol, pre-diabetes and diabetes. These are insidious conditions and can be present without symptoms.

• This is often a very stressful time in life as you are often starting to take care of elderly parents and are having increased life expenses, like children going to college. A lot of people express concerns about problems with work stress and sometimes start to have problems with relationships and divorce. For many people, however, this is a good time in life because you have a lot of wisdom under your belt and are much more comfortable with yourself than you were in your 20s or 30s. This can be a very liberating time in life for a lot of people. People have come into their own, navigate through life better, making intentional life decisions and can advocate for themselves and family through life challenges.

- This also starts to be the time in life where you start to be more comfortable with your own mortality, especially as friends and family start to have medical issues that are serious or fatal. Often many people start to come to the primary care physician at this time in life when they start to realize their own mortality and they decide to make a concerted effort to do preventive health things and have better control of chronic medical issues that they have been diagnosed with previously.

- Many people often embark on second careers, pursue further education related to their current job, or completely switch career paths during this stage of life. This change often brings a sense of invigoration and renewed enthusiasm.

- This is a very busy time of life between this decade and the next decade, and I often have to encourage patients not to forget about keeping their physical, medical and mental health in mind. It is very easy to let 10 years slip away and not keep up with medical issues (or ignore medical issues and symptoms that you are able to) and find that these conditions have gotten out of control. This is a decade that I meet a lot of patients who have come into the primary care office to re-establish care to get up-to-date on their healthcare because they have missed preventive care milestones like getting blood pressure checked, getting recommended Pap tests (cervical cancer screening), mammograms (breast cancer screening), colonoscopies (colon cancer screening), individualized disease screenings, depression and anxiety screening and getting labs done to screen for high cholesterol and diabetes. Many people find that their blood pressure is high when it didn't used to be. This is a decade where these silent issues can be going on while life is very busy. If you have not had any medical issues that are symptomatic enough to get you into a physician's office in your 30s, this is a time where the silent issues can start to manifest themselves. I often see patients in this age group where mild renal insufficiency (kidney disease) starts.

- This is the age group where chronic obesity starts to manifest its effects with chronic back pain, knee pain, ankle, and leg swelling. With increasing weight gain, the ability to tolerate daily activities and exercise decreases. Being short of breath doing housework and going up and down stairs are signs that your weight has gone beyond what is recommended for you and underlying, degenerative joint, heart or lung disease may be present.

AGE 51–60

- This is the time in life where people are often at the peak of their job, career or vocation and start to look forward to winding down with going to work every day. With the 2020 pandemic well underway, many people may be able to extend the time they work in life now with remote work opportunities being greatly expanded.
- This is also a time where people often express their desire to maintain their health, so they have some health and energy after anticipated retirement. People start to look forward to spending more time with family.

- This also can be a time where people who have not kept up with their medical issues previously in life start to have more serious problems. This is a time in life where it is very important to focus on minimizing the complications of chronic diseases that affect the cardiovascular system like diabetes, hypertension, and high blood pressure to minimize the risk of heart attack, stroke, cardiovascular eye disease and peripheral vascular disease. Preventing or having good control of these diseases can prevent or delay the onset of dementia and cognitive decline later in life.

- Many people in this decade have started to get diagnosed with malignancies like prostate cancer, colon cancer and breast cancer, but many people can be diagnosed in earlier stages where they can go through diagnosis and treatment and continue to progress to the next decades in life.

- This is the decade when orthopedic procedures start to increase with people getting back, hip and knee surgeries for painful degenerative disease (arthritis).

- Satisfactory sexual function is still desired at this time in life. In fact, having an active and satisfactory sex life is important to have across the decades. There are often medical conditions that can affect sexual function where changes in sexual function are the first sign of these disorders. In addition, inadequate control of many underlying medical conditions and/or medications used to treat these conditions can also affect sexual function. Treatment of undiagnosed medical conditions, improved control of medical conditions and making medications changes, if needed, can improve or solve sexual problems.

Psychological issues can also cause changes in sexual function and these conditions can be addressed as well. Any problems with sexual desire and sexual function should be discussed with your doctor.

AGES 61–70

- I see a lot of people in this age group that are either aging gracefully, retired and trying to enjoy life or becoming increasingly burdened with chronic medical issues, with an increase of taking medication, seeing specialists and getting diagnostic testing for evaluating symptoms and for chronic disease management.

- People often start to have more problems with muscle related back pain and joint issues that may have started developing the decade before. Unfortunately, chronic pain musculoskeletal conditions have to be managed with regularly assessing the risk and benefit of taking medications for chronic pain from arthritic/degenerative joint disease in the hips, knees, spine and other joints. These degenerative conditions cause increased problems and pain with walking and supportive walking devices (cane, walker, wheelchair) may start to be needed in this and the next decade.

- This is a time in life where role reversal starts and the caregiver to cared-for dynamic changes between parent and child. Older patients' home life and health care is increasingly being supervised or managed by adult children. Honestly, it is usually a daughter or daughter-in-law. Many patients in this age group, if they have had chronic medical or psychological issues earlier in life, have already had a deterioration in their health, such that they may no longer be living alone or may already be in a residential care facility (assisted living facility, nursing facility, or long-term care facility.)

- This is the time in life where often problems with bladder control can start in both men and women and these issues must be addressed.

- People begin to be even more comfortable discussing their own mortality and start talking to friends and family about their wishes (medical and financial) in the event of death, illness, or disability. (See section on Advanced Directives).

- This is the time of life where it begins to be important to have friend and family support with daily activities (housework, yard work, activities of daily living, money management). People start to rely more heavily on this support and find challenges with managing their lives when the support network is not there or was not developed in previous decades in life. Serious medical issues often lead to admissions to assisted living facilities and nursing homes when care at home becomes infeasible due to the amount of care that is needed or the lack of support at home to provide the appropriate care. Often adult children are still working away from home and grandchildren may still be too young to provide care when daycare is needed. (The 2020 pandemic altered this dynamic in many ways). Community senior day care services are very helpful to provide daycare when assisted living residency or nursing home care is not yet needed or desired.

- Staying mentally and physically active at this time helps to prevent future anxiety and depression. It also helps prevent trouble sleeping. Staying active with something as simple as walking daily can help muscle strength and prevent falls and lessen injury with falls.

AGE 71–80

- There are many patients in this age group who still do very well even though they may have chronic medical issues. They still maintain their cognitive function and ability to remain independent and have lives that are still meaningful to them. Many in this group still travel to visit friends and family. Many are still driving safely. They use cell phones and the internet and are still very involved in using social media, keeping up with current events, using health care patient portals to refill medications, communicate with their health care professions and navigate our health care system, such as it is, using these modalities.
- Patients in this age group may still have a spouse/life partner and I have noticed that over time, they increasingly come to depend on each other for support and care. There are many people in this age group who are still very active with exercise and sexual activity.
- Many people may start to have more challenging problems with their cognitive function and start to have the onset of dementia which can be primary or secondary/ multi factorial in nature. Most people who have a decline in cognitive (thinking) function is not due to Alzheimer's Dementia, which is a specific type of dementia, among

many types of dementia. Many people have a decline in cognitive function due to inactivity, depression/anxiety and vascular (causes that come from diseases that affect the arteries that give blood to the brain) like high blood pressure, diabetes, high cholesterol and kidney disease. Many need more assistance with using cell phones and the internet to use health care patient portals to refill medications, communicate with their health care professions and navigate our health care system.

- Injury from falls is a large risk in this age group and in the next decade, often having serious or lethal consequences. Living conditions should be regularly assessed for slip and fall hazards like rugs, uneven floors and furniture and objects in walkways in the home. Having adequate lighting at night is necessary to prevent falls while going to the bathroom.

AGE 81–90

- Very often, patients in this age group are now living with an adult child or grandchild or both where the adults are very much involved in their activities of daily living (meal preparation, grooming and personal care, managing finances, washing clothes, etc.) and home care if they are still living at home and not in a residential facility. There are many, however, that still live independently, alone or with a significant other in the same age group, with loved ones living very close by. Most have at least one chronic medical condition and take at least 1-3 daily medications.

- Many have trouble with bladder and bowel incontinence, but many still do not. Typically, trouble with incontinence is the consequence of not being able to get to the bathroom fast enough, rather than an actual bowel or bladder problem. By now, many are living in one-story homes or live on one level and use bedside commodes to manage this problem.

BE AN ACTIVE PARTICIPANT
IN YOUR HEALTH:

BEING HEALTHY AND
FIT IS A LIFESTYLE.

8

How to Help Your Doctor Help You

*B*EING AN ACTIVE PARTICIPANT IN YOUR OWN HEALTH will give you the best opportunity to maintain health and prevent disease. Getting recommended evaluations, doing home self-monitoring of medical conditions and how you feel can empower you to care for yourself and minimize the need for you and your doctor to have to do "heavy lifting" medically with you in the future. The more you keep track of your health action items and preventive health gaps, the more you can optimize your health to promote overall well-being and disease prevention over time. Furthermore, being aware of and having documentation of your medical history and previous medical evaluations will enable your doctor to provide better care for you.

PREVENTIVE CARE

- Get a preventive health visit once a year. In addition to having good eating and exercise habits, keeping up with recommended preventive health testing and recommended screenings is the best thing you can do to prevent illnesses that we have the ability to find early and do something about.

- Get a flu shot every fall. "Influenza (flu) is a contagious respiratory illness caused by influenza viruses. It can cause mild to severe illness. Serious outcomes of flu infection can result in hospitalization or death. Some people, such as older people, young children, and people with certain health conditions, are at high risk of serious flu complications. There are two main types of influenza (flu) virus: Types A and B. The influenza A and B viruses that routinely spread in people (human influenza viruses) are responsible for seasonal flu epidemics each year. The best way to prevent flu is by getting vaccinated each year." Getting a flu shot is recommended for all adults. (https://www.cdc.gov/flu/about/index.html-https://www.cdc.gov/mmwr/volumes/69/rr/rr6908a1.htm) Per the CDC, "influenza can be associated with serious illnesses, hospitalizations, and deaths, particularly among older adults, very young children, pregnant women, and persons of all ages with certain chronic medical conditions. Influenza also is an important cause of missed work and school." Check with your doctor to discuss any medical conditions you may have that make you vulnerable to suffering from serious illness from the respiratory virus that causes influenza.
- Get other vaccines that are recommended for you. The general recommendations for adult vaccinations are detailed in the previous section, "Health is Not About Ordering tests." You should discuss what vaccinations

are recommended for you with your doctor. If you are traveling abroad, there may be other vaccinations that are needed for entrance into other countries. The CDC website is a good resource for this information. You can get up to date information about vaccination requirements for the countries that you are planning to travel to at https://wwwnc.cdc.gov/travel/destinations/list.

- Know your medical insurance plan coverage for preventive health visits. Many medical insurance plans only pay for medical visits when a medical diagnosis or condition is addressed. Conversely, some insurance plans only pay for preventive health visits and if there is a medical issue addressed at the visit, the insurance will not pay for that visit. Sometimes you may need to make two separate visits to address a medical issue separate from a visit where only preventive health issues are addressed. Be sure to contact your insurance company to find out how your medical insurance plan works. Your physician will not typically know this unless you inform them.

YOUR DOCTOR VISITS

- Know your copayment requirements of your insurance plan and make sure that your medical insurance is active before your doctor visit. This will prevent the need to re-schedule your appointment.
- Arrive or log-on 15–30 minutes early to your doctor's office or video visits. This facilitates completing pre-visit tasks (front office or online check-in, checking blood pressure in the office or at home, reviewing medications,

doing in-office testing, giving pre-ordered immunizations, etc.) so that your actual time with the doctor can
be more efficiently used. Fill out pre-visit questionnaires
on the patient portal before your visit, when applicable.

- For your first visit with a doctor, especially when choosing a new primary care doctor, bring any and all previous
medical records, medication bottles, preventive health
test results, immunizations, surgeries, names of specialists,
diagnoses to the first visit so your medical history can be
reviewed. Contact all of your previous doctors before or
right after the first visit with your new doctor. The sooner
your medical records can be reviewed, the smoother the
transition of your medical care. Know and keep records of
the names of all the specialists you have seen in the past
and are currently. You should know why you saw them
and what was the outcome of those evaluations.

- Know what immunizations you have had in your life and
the date of when they were given.

- Keep records and know the date of your last wellness/
preventive health visit, Pap test with HPV co-testing,
colonoscopy, mammogram, immunizations, diabetic eye
exam, diabetic foot exam and last time you had your cholesterol and blood sugar checked.

- Know and keep an ongoing list of all of the surgeries
(even childhood procedures) and procedures that you've
had, including who did the procedure, when you had the
procedure and why it was done.

- If you've had a hysterectomy, know if you have had the
entire uterus removed or if your cervix is still in place. It
is useful to know if your ovaries were also removed or not
with the uterus. Knowing what organs are still in place

informs your doctor about what screening tests need to be recommended for you.

- Keep a folder (paper or electronic/digital) of all your medical documents and have them available when you meet a new doctor.

- Let your primary care doctor know about any medications you have been prescribed by any of your specialists and let your specialist(s) know about any medication changes that you have had at every visit.

- Know and record your family history. Medical conditions in your family tree may affect you greatly. It is very important to ask your parents, siblings and grandparents about their medical issues. Encourage them to go to the doctor to get their recommended screening and checks and communicate their medical issues with you. Write down this information to share with your doctor. Knowing this family information may come in handy if you need to assist them with managing their own medical care at a later date.

If you are assisting an elderly family member with their new doctor's visit, you will need to gather their medical information for them. I often have adult children of patients that don't know their parent or family member's medical history, and this makes it difficult taking care of them because that patient was previously able to manage their own health care. When their ability to do this declines, their adult children are often unfamiliar with their medical history. I've had adult children of patients who were shocked to learn their parents had significant conditions like cancer, heart disease and kidney disease. I will also point out here that it is good practice to share your medical conditions with people who may need to care for you later on in life. Often parents move in with their adult children after living independently in another state. Gathering medical information is more challenging in these cases, but necessary. With the widespread use of EMR's, (electronic medical record) though, many large institutions allow electronic interfaces to pull medical records into the chart if the patient authorizes this function.

- Bring all your medication bottles, prescription and over the counter (allergy medication, aspirin, cold medications, eye drops, pain medication, etc.), to every doctor visit to make sure that each doctor you see can review everything you are taking, including supplements, vitamins, creams, and inhalers. Non-prescription medication can interact with other medications and your doctor cannot evaluate the safety of your medications without full disclosure. Even NSAID's (non-steroidal anti-inflammatory drugs) can have side effects, like raising blood pressure, causing stomach ulcers, and kidney damage. Have all of this available and in front of you with video visits as well. Often patients have medications that have been discontinued and have medications which were incorrectly filled by their pharmacy. This is why having just a medication list at your doctor's visit is inadequate.

- Sign up for the patient portal if your doctor and/or health care system has this service with an electronic medical record (EMR). Using the patient portal allows you to be a more active participant in your own health care. Using a patient portal can be an invaluable resource to communicate with your doctor with questions and concerns, to request prescription refills, see your medication list and add new medications prescribed elsewhere. The patient portal can help you keep up with all appointment related activities, including past, present and upcoming appointments. You can review your problem/diagnosis list and preventive health and immunization recommendations and gaps. You can see and review many of your test results and your actual physician notes about you in your patient portal immediately. This is a way to review what was discussed at your doctor's visit. 21st Century Cures Act federal legislation went into effect April 2021 to allow "easy access to your health records puts you in control of decisions regarding your health and well-being. You can monitor your health conditions better, understand and stay on track with treatment plans, and find and fix errors in your record." (https://www.healthit.gov/topic/patient-access-health-records/patient-access-health-records and https://www.healthit.gov/curesrule/overview/about-oncs-cures-act-final-rule)

Be mindful that an immediate test result release to you means that your results may not have been reviewed by your doctor at the time that you view them. In addition, patient notes are full of medical terminology and acronyms that you may not understand. Patient portals are also a secure way for you to upload documents to be a part of your medical record for your doctor to review. Some EMR's allow you to organize your health information by storing medical documents for only your view in your patient portal. In addition, if you are seeing several doctors who use a shared EMR, all your doctors can see your medical records. Patient portal information can be easily accessed on a desktop, computer, laptop, tablet or smartphone.

In addition, with the widespread use of EMR's, many large health institutions and health systems allow electronic interfaces to pull medical records into the chart from outside institutions and systems if the patient authorizes this function. Often, United States Department of Defense medical records interface well with certain EMR's, if allowed, and many states have immunization registries and local hospital, radiology facility and regional medical record databases that you authorize (or can decline) your medical information to be able to be accessed when you receive care at participating health care facilities, hospitals, medical offices and emergency departments.

- Take a notebook with you to your doctor's visits so you can keep notes. There are many things you and your doctor will discuss during your visit, and you may forget some things once the visit is over. Review and save documents you are given during your visit for you to review later.

- Record questions for your doctor in between visits so you don't forget important questions that you want to ask. Everything on your list may not need to be addressed all in one visit but keeping a record of your questions to review at each can help you help your doctor prioritize your concerns to address at future meetings.

- Respond to and/or read/review all correspondence (voicemail, cell phone text, patient portal, postal mail) from your doctor or doctor's office. We've found that patients are very busy and do not always answer telephone calls during business hours, so many times trying to communicate with people by telephone is not effective. We rely on the secure forms of communication detailed above to relay medical information beyond trying to catch a patient with a direct conversation by telephone. By the way, e-mail is not a safe way to communicate medical information.

- If you have high blood pressure, check your blood pressure daily and bring your blood pressure machine to your doctor's visit so it can be checked for accuracy, appropriate arm cuff size and to make sure you are using it properly. Blood pressure should be checked with a machine with an arm cuff and not with a cuff around the wrist or finger. You should record your daily blood pressure readings on paper or enter them into your physician patient portal. Sending blood pressure readings in between visits (dropping them off to the office or sending your readings electronically using your patient portal allows your doctor to review your readings in between visits and intervene with changes in your care, if needed). Most digital blood pressure machines now have a memory that saves 60-90 blood pressure readings to review with your doctor. Change the batteries in your blood pressure machine every 3 months to make sure you are getting the best accuracy from your blood pressure machine.

- If you have diabetes, check your blood sugar daily and bring your glucose meter to each doctor visit to review your diabetes control. Many EMR's allow you to enter (manually and sometimes automatically from a device) and record your blood glucose (blood sugar) readings for your doctor to review (and intervene, if needed) in between visits. Many doctor's offices now have devices to upload your glucose meter readings into the EMR.

- Make an appointment to follow up with your doctor when recommended right after your visit before leaving the office or on the same day you have a video visit. Patient portals typically allow you to make appointment requests and some even allow you to schedule your own future appointments. Having a future appointment ensures that you do not have gaps in your care and that you follow up in the timeframe that your doctor has recommended.

- No news is not always good news. Make sure you get verbal or written (electronic or on paper) test results for all tests ordered. I have reviewed many medical records for new patients coming to me where patients report that abnormal test results were never communicated to them. "If you don't hear anything from me, everything is OK," is not an acceptable way to know what your test results are. Using your patient portal to see test results is a good way to keep up with the findings of testing done. If test results have not been communicated to you, in any form, make an appointment to discuss your test results with the doctor who ordered the test.

The most common test abnormality that a patient tells me they were unaware of after I review previous medical records is an abnormal PAP test (cervical cancer screening test). Being unaware of an abnormal PAP test can have dire consequences for a woman and subsequently, her family. On more than a few occasions, I've had new patients who've had an abnormal PAP test from their last exam say that they weren't notified of the results. Therefore, the interval for follow up on the abnormal PAP test was missed. Unfortunately for some, their repeat PAP showed progression of the abnormality to a worse stage of the pre-cancerous cervical abnormality prompting referral to GYN for further evaluation and treatment.

- If you have a doctor who you feel is not listening to you or is not responsive to your needs, consider changing doctors. Make sure you get all of your medical records from the old doctor as soon as you know you are changing your care to someone else.

YOUR MEDICATIONS

- Be willing to advocate for yourself for insurance plan denials for medications and diagnostic testing. Call your insurance company to find out about the appeals process for denials of payment for medications and procedures. Don't give up if your insurance will not pay for something requested by you or your doctor. Often medical insurance company payment denial decisions can be reversed by appealing the decision.
- Request medication refills at least one week before your prescription is due to run out. Delays can occur with medication refills, and you don't want to risk running out of your regular medications.
- Let your doctor's office know when your preferred pharmacy changes or when your mailing address, telephone number, or e-mail address changes. Incorrect pharmacy and contact information are a significant source of delays in fulfilling prescription refill requests and following up on patient communication.

- Keeping in mind that doctor's offices are busy, give yourself enough time for a response when you need a referral, order, or a letter written. Please let your doctor or pharmacist know if you ever get prescription pills you do not recognize or have a question about. Don't assume that what you have been given is correct. Pharmacies often change manufacturers, such that your pills may look different, even if it's the same medication. You should clarify this with the pharmacy beforehand.

- Be familiar with how to get your insurance pharmacy information from your medical insurance company. Many insurance plans have booklets that can be mailed to you or have medication formulary information available online. Be ready to contact your insurance company about alternative medications when a medication that you are prescribed is denied for payment or coverage.

- Contact your doctor immediately if you have a problem taking a medication, getting a medication filled at your pharmacy, seeing a specialist that you have been referred to or getting testing done that has been ordered for you. The doctor and/or office staff can be very helpful in helping you get medications, schedule appointments for specialists, and diagnostic testing.

- Take all medication as prescribed. Do not change how you take your medication before communicating with your doctor first. Changing your medication dosing may not be safe. If your medication dosing needs to be changed, your doctor can tell you how to do it safely.

HOW DO YOU FEEL?

- It's a good habit to journal how you feel every day, or at least weekly. Patients often forget symptoms because they may be minor or fleeting, but nonetheless important when put together, especially if there is a pattern to the symptoms that are not apparent if the symptom(s) are infrequent. Keeping a diary of your daily symptoms in a journal to review with your doctor is quite useful in diagnosing a problem that you are having.
- Keep a food diary. Symptoms are often related to meals or eating certain foods so keeping a diary of what you eat can help your doctor find the cause of many symptoms.
- Get enough sleep. Many medical conditions are caused or exacerbated by not getting enough restful sleep.
- Don't ignore symptoms, even symptoms that seem minor. Always let your doctor know about any new symptoms you are having, especially a symptom you cannot explain easily.

As previously mentioned, avoid looking up symptoms on the Internet. More often than not, searching symptoms on the internet in an effort to diagnose the cause of the symptoms leads to unnecessary anxiety and worry.

- Keep track of how much coffee you drink, how many cigarettes you smoke per day, and how many alcohol drinks you drink per day or per week. It is helpful to be able to quantify these things for your doctor, so your doctor can make recommendations about modification of these things to help improve your health and also make disease screening and testing recommendations based on these social habits.

- If you ever get an insect bite or, in particular a tick bite, put the tick in a plastic bag or container, because it can be sent to the lab for identification. Tick and insect borne diseases can be more easily diagnosed or ruled out if the insect can be exactly identified. Many patients are concerned about getting Lyme Disease from insect bites, but fortunately most insect bites that patients have are not caused by the specific tick that carries the organism that causes Lyme Disease.

- Take a picture of any skin conditions. Often skin conditions will be resolved by the time you get to see the doctor in person or by video visit and a picture can often help with diagnosing a cause.

- If you ever have a sore throat, take a flashlight, and look in the back of your throat and take note of what you see so you can describe it to your doctor. Take a picture if you can. This is very helpful considering the cause of a sore throat.

- After bowel movements, always look at your stool and take note of any changes (color and appearance, i.e., loose, formed, shape), including the presence of blood. In addition, observing the location of blood in stool is useful in determining the source of the blood (blood on top of the stool, blood mixed in the stool or blood in the toilet water) and a possible diagnosis.

9

Your First Visit

*T*HE FIRST VISIT WITH YOUR DOCTOR IS THE FOUNDATION of your future care. The more information your doctor has, the better your care will be. These are all questions you should be prepared to answer or have the information ready for your new doctor to begin your care. Each question that is asked at your initial visit with your doctor has a medical reason to be asked so that your current health status can be assessed and current and future medical recommendations can be made. Having all of this information on the first visit is the best way to have a smooth transition of your care.

I had a new patient that came to me to establish care. She arrived with none of her medical records and couldn't remember the names of specialists she had seen previously. I reviewed what I could of her medical history and requested the medical records from her previous physicians. Review of her medical records revealed she didn't remember many critical aspects of her previous care, including significant diagnosis and surgeries. This prompted me to have the patient and her daughter schedule a follow up appointment to communicate the extreme urgency that was needed to her care that was not apparent at our first visit. I reviewed her medical conditions and explained to both the significance of her medical history with respect to how she should be eating, smoking cessation and testing and referrals that I needed to order immediately to continue the evaluation of her current concerns that her previous physicians had started.

Be prepared to tell your story from the womb until the day of your visit. Do not forget about medical issues during childhood or adolescence. Medical issues occurring early in life often have significant ramifications well into adulthood.

Some questions for consideration:

- If you are under twenty-five-years old, who was your pediatrician? Do you have your immunization records? Do you know your blood type? Do you know your status of sickle cell trait or not?
- When did you last see your last primary care doctor and what was their name? How long were you seeing that doctor?
- Why are you changing your primary care doctor?
- What are the names of all medications that you take? What are you taking them for?
- What symptoms are bothering you?
- What is your family history, especially of your parents, siblings? What was their diagnosis and how old were they when they were diagnosed?
- What do you eat on a regular basis?
- What kind of exercise do you do and how often do you do it?
- When was your last flu shot, shingles vaccine, tetanus shot, pneumonia vaccination, COVID 19 vaccination,

eye exam, dental visit, podiatrist visit, dermatologist visit?

- When is the last time you were tested for HIV, hepatitis B, hepatitis C, syphilis, Chlamydia, gonorrhea? What were the results?
- How do you currently protect yourself against sexually transmitted diseases?
- Are you doing anything to not be pregnant or not father children?
- Are you currently trying to get pregnant? Are you using any aids to get pregnant (ovulation kit, taking temperature)?
- Do you have Advance Directives or a Living Will written down? Do you have Durable Power of Attorney of Health Care (someone to make medical decisions for you in the event that you cannot make decisions for yourself?)
- How are you feeling mentally and psychologically? Are you having any thoughts of suicide or symptoms of anxiety or depression?
- Do you have a history of abuse, neglect, or exploitation?
- When was your last visit to a dermatologist for a skin cancer screening or assessment of skin conditions, skin lesions, or moles?
- When was the last time you had a preventive health visit?
- When was the last time any blood was drawn, who ordered the tests, for what reason and what were the results?
- When did you have to visit an urgent care or emergency room? For what reason? Where did you go/what facility? What was evaluated? What were the results or outcome of the evaluation?
- What specialists have you seen, for what reason, and what were the results of the evaluations?

- Do you currently see any specialists, for what conditions and what current treatments are being done?
- What have you had images (x-rays, CT scan, MRI's ultrasounds) taken for in your life, what body parts, where were they done and for what reason? What were the results?
- Have you ever had a heart stress test, echocardiogram, cardiac catheterization, or any other type of heart testing?
- Have you ever smoked? At what age did you start smoking, when did you quit smoking? On average, over the course of being a smoker, how much did you smoke (packs per day)?
- If you are or have been a smoker, have you ever had lung cancer screening with an annual low dose CT scan of the chest?
- If you are a man and /or have been a smoker, have you ever had abdominal aortic aneurysm screening with an ultrasound of the abdominal aorta?

QUESTIONS FOR WOMEN

- When was your last menstrual period?
- Have you ever been pregnant? If so, how many total times you were pregnant?
- How did you deliver and did you have any medical issues or complications with pregnancy or delivery?
- Have you ever taken any female hormones for any reason (pregnancy prevention, trying to get pregnant, for acne treatment, for irregular bleeding, or not having periods, for heaving bleeding)?

- Are you having or have you had problems with periods, how often do have periods, how long is your period?
- When was your last Pap and HPV test, last mammogram, last bone density test?
- How old were you when your first period started?
- Do you have any problems with your periods (nausea, vomiting, headaches, diarrhea, mood swings, heavy bleeding, back pain)?
- Do you do a monthly self-breast exam (7-10 days after menses, if you are still having periods?)

10

How to Describe a Symptom / What Matters in a Symptom?

*I*F YOUR DOCTOR DOES NOT GET THE STORY RIGHT ABOUT your symptoms(s), your evaluation may go down the wrong path. You should do your best to describe specifics about your symptoms, not leaving out any detail, no matter how insignificant you think it is. Sometimes the simplest detail of a symptom can make the difference between making the correct diagnosis or not. Any symptom matters.

Writing down symptoms (and taking pictures of skin conditions, lumps and bumps, etc.) is very helpful in helping to figure out what is causing a symptom or causing how you are feeling. I encourage patients to write a daily journal of "Symptom and Food Diary." This allows you to document how you are feeling, especially if symptoms do not occur very often. When patients are in the doctor's often trying to explain a symptom, they often omit important symptoms and details of how they have been feeling. A journal allows you to document how a symptom is occurring, when it is occurring, what is going on in your life at the time it occurs, what other symptoms accompany the symptom, and what you have been eating that may affect the symptom. By writing it down, patients often find the symptoms are occurring less or more frequently than they remember. Symptom journaling also allows you to see if there is a pattern to symptoms over time.

Other questions for consideration:

- When did the symptom start? 1 month ago? 1 year ago? 10 years ago? Many symptoms start a long time ago, even from childhood, and persist over many weeks, months or even a year. You need to tell your doctor about when the symptoms started, even in its mildest form. This still matters and may be significant.
- What does it feel like? Is it sharp? Dull? Burning? Stabbing? Shooting? Move from one body area to another?
- How often does it happen? Once a day? Once a week? Once a month? It is helpful to keep a diary of symptoms, especially a symptom that happens infrequently. There may be a pattern that becomes apparent when you write down a symptom that happens infrequently.
- What makes it better or makes it go away?
- Is it associated with something you eat or when you do not eat?
- How long does it last?
- What symptoms occur at the same time with it?
- Does it happen at any particular time of day or location? In the morning? At home? At work? Outside only? While driving? With exercise? With certain movements of body positions?

A thorough review of symptoms you are feeling or physical signs that you see on your body is the most important part of the physician visit after the history. Patients often forget about symptoms, so I frequently ask them to review a list of symptoms to see if there are any others present that could aid in the evaluation.

Review of this list of symptoms by category helps me see how a patient feels and helps to prioritize current and future evaluations:

GENERAL

- Tired with activity
- Decreased appetite
- Chills
- Fever
- Night sweats
- Confusion/ disorientation
- Dizziness
- Drooling
- Edema/swelling in body/legs
- Fainting
- Fatigue/unusual tiredness
- Feeling feverish
- Itching
- Itchy eyes
- Sleeping problems
- Unusual weakness
- Weight gain/loss
- Loss of height
- Frequent falls

RESPIRATORY

- Cough
- Nasal stuffiness
- Rapid breathing
- Runny nose
- Shortness of breath
- Shortness of breath while lying down
- Waking up short of breath
- Loud snoring

- Sore throat
- Sneezing
- Throat clearing
- Wheezing
- Coughing up blood

GASTROINTESTINAL

- Problems eating
- Problems chewing
- Problems swallowing
- Belching
- Bloating
- Heartburn
- Frequent constipation
- Abdominal cramping
- Abdominal pain
- Frequent diarrhea
- Distention/belly full of air
- Flatulence/passing lots of gas
- Hemorrhoids
- Hiccoughing
- Losing control of stool
- Blood in stool/very dark or black stools
- Nausea
- Vomiting
- Vomiting blood

EAR, NOSE AND THROAT

- Decreased hearing/ hearing problems
- Earache/ear pain
- Ear discharge
- Hoarseness
- Nasal congestion
- Nosebleeds
- Ears ringing
- Stuffy nose
- Runny nose
- Sinus pain
- Sore throat

SKIN

- Change in skin color
- Dry skin
- Rashes
- Lumps, bumps, sores, boils or hives

HEART

- Chest pain/pressure at rest
- Chest pain/pressure with activity
- Pain in legs with walking
- Palpitations/feeling a fast heartbeat

URINE/BLADDER

- Not urinating at all
- Decreased urinating
- Dribbling of urine
- Burning/pain with urinating
- Urinating a lot
- Blood in urine
- Hesitation with urine coming out
- Leaking urine/losing control of urine coming out
- Urinating at night a lot
- Trouble urinating/decrease urine stream
- Urge to urinate a lot
- Frequent urinary tract infections

NERVES

- Weakness on one side of body
- Can't move one side of body
- Numbness/tingling
- Jerking with movements
- Tremors
- Change in feeling in any body part
- Change in speech
- Seizures
- Loss of consciousness

BRAIN

- Trouble concentrating
- Drowsiness
- Headaches
- Memory problems
- Eye problems
- Eye pain
- Eye redness
- Blurry vision
- Trouble seeing
- Eye discharge
- Seeing double
- Bright lights bothering eyes
- Yellow eyes or yellow skin

PSYCHIATRIC

- Anxiety or nervousness
- Panic attacks
- Depression/feeling sad
- Mood changes/mood swings
- Thinking of things that are not real
- Seeing things that are not real
- Being over excited
- Being paranoid

- Being overly afraid of something
- Thinking of suicide
- Drinking too much alcohol
- Taking illegal drugs or prescription drug abuse
- Memory problems

ENDOCRINE/HORMONES

- Feeling too cold
- Feeling hungry too much
- Thirstiness
- Feeling too hot

BLOOD/LYMPH NODES

- Bleeding/bruising more easily
- Enlarged lymph nodes
- Swollen glands in neck or groin

MUSCULAR/SLEEP SYMPTOMS

- Back pain
- Joint pain
- Joint stiffness
- Joint swelling
- Muscle cramps
- Restless legs in bed
- Loud snoring
- Muscle pain
- Pain in legs with walking

SEXUAL FUNCTION

- Decreased sexual desire
- Problems with orgasms
- Pain with sex
- Discharge from nipples

FEMALE

- Vaginal discharge
- Vaginal itching
- Change in vaginal odor
- Problems with periods
- Hot flashes

MALE

- Decreased erections
- Discharge from penis
- Lumps, bumps or skin changes on the penis or scrotum

11

Pressuring Your Doctor

$\mathcal{I}$ HAD AN INTERESTING DISCUSSION WITH A PATIENT THAT followed me to my new practice location to continue her care. She started the visit telling me she was going to follow my instructions and stop "bullying you this time." I jotted down this point when she said to me that she was going to focus on following my recommendations, even the recommendations that she doesn't like, primarily with respect to changing her eating habits. She felt she was not accomplishing her health goals over the course of our doctor-patient relationship, and she wanted to make changes to do so.

When I asked her what she meant by her statement, she said she previously tried to aggressively "bully" me to get what she wanted or thought she needed. She felt she decided what she wanted for her health and didn't want to listen to my explanations when I declined to prescribe medication or order a test that I felt was not needed or warranted and/or wanted to prescribe medications, treatments, and diet recommendations that I felt she would benefit from. I understood what she meant, and she was not talking about asking for pain medication, narcotic medication, or medications that patients use to "get high" or for euphoria (drug seeking behavior).

I have often felt "bullied" by patients who wanted me to prescribe medications that I didn't think were safe or necessary. When I asked her, "Why do people bully their doctors like this?" She said, "People look up and find things (medications, devices, treatments, testing) on the internet and think they know more than the doctor about what they need for their health." I thought about what she said, and I agreed with her assessment. I think patients have access to so much medical information and then arrive at the medical office with their perception and strong feelings about what they want or need.

Insisting that your doctor prescribe a treatment or medication that they have reasoned is unsafe or unwarranted for you can have negative consequences. I told her that doctors are people too, and often do not push back or decline these requests when patients "bully" them and this causes patients to often end up taking medications for conditions they don't have, taking medications they don't need and/or getting unnecessary diagnostic testing. I explained to her that pressuring a doctor into giving what the patient wants often leads to the prescription of medications that are unnecessary and can put the patient at risk of having medication side effects from a medication that is not needed or recommended. In addition, ordering tests that are not recommended puts the patient at risk for getting false-positive test results which can cause anxiety, especially when tests are ordered without a clear reason and just to satisfy the patient.

Often patients come to the doctor with an agenda that has nothing to do with improving or at least maintaining their health. This can be dangerous to the patient. This is even more common than people just simply wanting medications that alter their mental status (drug seeking behavior). Sometimes patients want medications to accomplish a cosmetic concern, like wanting to get rid of changes on the skin or something on the body that is visible. Recommending a treatment for a cosmetic reason first requires finding the underlying cause of the condition before recommending a treatment or medication that just masks what is seen on the body externally.

The most common request for a new or refill prescription that I receive is the request for diuretics (water pills) for leg and/or ankle swelling. I have had countless patients ask for a refill on a diuretic that was prescribed by their previous physician and the patient reports that the cause for the leg and ankle swelling was never evaluated, which often their previous medical records confirm. I do not prescribe or refill diuretics unless there is a medical reason to do so. Diuretics have many uses but can have side effects. Therefore, just like with any prescription, there should be a specific medical reason for taking a diuretic. In these cases, I review previous medical records and/or investigate the reason for the swelling. In every case, I always find a reason for the leg and ankle swelling (serious and not as serious) and there are only a very small number of conditions that I find that warrants continuing a diuretic.

Sometimes, a patient may desire a medication that they've seen someone else taking, without understanding that the other person's medical background and condition may necessitate that specific medication. When I am presented with these requests, I review the patient's concern to see if the medication in question would be appropriate or not.

When a request like this is made, patients are often very receptive when they are allowed to expound upon what they are concerned about. But this is after I take a detailed medical history and review of symptoms and then explain what I think maybe going on. I also recommend, if applicable, what diagnostic testing may help to further evaluate the symptoms and/or what specialists may be helpful. I then explain why the test, medication or treatment that is being requested is not appropriate for them. This often may take 1-3 visits after having reviewed past and current symptoms with the patient and having reviewed previous medical records.

Explaining my plan for evaluation to address the concern helps to allay the patient's anxiety about symptoms or conditions they are experiencing. Patients are often unaware of the appropriate method for evaluating physical or psychological symptoms. Evaluating a symptom or concern is best done by using a systematic, scientific, evidence-based approach such that the plan of action discussed between the doctor and the patient can have the best chance of proceeding to a meaningful evaluation and conclusion. Diagnostic testing results are difficult to interpret if the reason for ordering the testing is not as clear as possible.

We are in an environment where patients have access to medical information, which is empowering for them and allows patients to be better informed about medical issues and advocates of their own health. However, sometimes what patients want and/or think they need is often not appropriate or beneficial. Patients are often focused on ordering tests instead of understanding the significance of having doctors do a complete medical history and examination, if needed, to appropriately order what testing may be needed to get to the root cause of a potential medical problem or condition.

I try to educate patients to change their way of thinking about ordering tests. Ordering a test without being clear on the reason why you are ordering the test or what you are going to do about any of the result possibilities makes the result interpretation vague and often not useful.

Even after going through a detailed medical history, review of symptoms, explanation of the diagnostic plan, patients want what they want based on what someone told them, what they saw on television or read somewhere, which may not apply to them. This is a negative consequence, especially of direct-to-consumer advertising for medications. I explain to patients that often the medications they are seeing on television or reading about are not new medications, but often more expensive "me-too" drugs whose comparable and cheaper alternatives are the same but are not advertised in the media anymore.

I recently had a patient request a weight loss medication that she saw on television. I had never heard of the medication, so I looked it up. I found the medication had recently been released to the market to use for diabetes and weight loss. (There are several medications that we prescribed for weight loss and to treat diabetes as well). This medication is very similar to drugs that have already been in use for several years, and I was able to explain the uses of this class of medication and the implication of using the medication for her specifically. I directed her to check with her insurance company to find out which of the medications, if any, was covered for her, as any of them would be useful to try for weight loss (in conjunction with healthy eating and regular exercise). I then prescribed an older medication in the same class, after she found out from her insurance company that the medication she asked about was not covered anyway. A new medication in a class is not necessarily superior to older medications of the same class.

The American Board of Internal Medicine's (ABIM) Choosing Wisely is a good online resource to look at what testing and diagnostic studies have evidence to support (and NOT support) consideration for various medical conditions and preventive health recommendations. Choosing Wisely is an initiative of the ABIM Foundation that seeks to advance a national dialogue on avoiding unnecessary medical tests, treatments, and procedures. (https://www.choosingwisely.org/our-mission/history/)

12

"I Want Everything Done."

WE ALL ARE ANXIOUS ABOUT DEVELOPING MEDICAL AND health conditions in the future. Sometimes a patient's fears of having a medical issue prompts them to tell me that they "want to be tested for everything." Similarly, I often get new patients who have made an appointment with me and want a current evaluation of their health and want to be "tested for everything".

I communicate to patients there is no such thing (and never really was such a thing) as getting "tested for everything." Unfortunately, for most medical issues that a person can have, we do not have the ability to diagnose early. This is often a difficult concept for patients to grasp because medical advances have progressed so far that there is so much we can now do in the medical field. However, there are many more medical conditions that we do not have a cure for, nor do we have diagnostic testing to find them early enough to do something about.

What is more important than getting "everything done" during an annual physical is making sure that you are up to date on your recommended preventive health screenings that have been detailed previously. Even though there is not a lot of scientific evidence for doing "the annual physical," I still think doing regular preventive health or wellness visits once a year is very useful to catch up on any symptoms that are bothering you, review your medical history and family history and make sure that preventive health items have been addressed, and complete preventive health gaps that exist. The most important part of the preventive health visit is reviewing what the patient is eating to make sure healthy eating is a daily part of the patient's lifestyle. Eating healthy is the best thing that anyone can do to improve or at least maintain health and prevent disease. In this country, cardiovascular disease is still a significant cause of morbidity and mortality and there is a lot of evidence that low-fat and more plant-based eating is helpful in preventing all types of cancers and helps in many autoimmune disorders.

Unfortunately, for men, there are only two cancers that we have a good way to find early. Primarily, this is colon cancer by starting colon cancer screening now at age 45. The second cancer is prostate cancer, however, the early diagnosis of prostate cancer that may become a future problem is challenging with the currently limited capability of the annual PSA test and digital rectal exam.

For women, there are only three cancers that we have good screening tests for. Colon cancer screening is also recommended for women starting at age 45. The annual mammogram starting at age 40 is recommended for breast cancer screening. The PAP test with HPV co-testing when recommended is good for cervical cancer screening with frequency decided upon depending on age and risk factors.

13

Ordering Tests

O RDERING TESTS OUTSIDE OF PREVENTIVE HEALTH
testing and screenings is based upon various patient factors,
including an individual's medical history, family history, medications, and any past or current symptoms. When ordering tests,
even a simple test, you should have a clear reason why the test
is being ordered. If the reason for ordering a test is not defined,
the meaning of the result will often be difficult to interpret. More
importantly, test result possibilities should always be considered
and discussed before ordering any tests. I find it useful to discuss
test result possibilities so the patient is educated about what the
next possible recommended steps will be with each possible test
result or outcome. After review of the possible test results or outcomes, particularly the undesirable test result outcome, many
patients decide they do not want the test being discussed because
they will not want to do the next stage of testing that will be recommended for the undesirable test result.

A good example of this is the discussion that I have with patients about whether to continue to get a mammogram (a test
done to screen for breast cancer) in a woman that has never been

diagnosed with breast cancer. There are well-defined ages where colon cancer screening (colonoscopy etc.) and cervical cancer screening (Pap test and HPV co-testing) should stop unless there is a specific reason to continue screening. However, it is less clear about what age to stop getting mammograms. (https://www. cancer.org/healthy/find-cancer-early/american-cancer-society-guidelines-for-the-early-detection-of-cancer.html), (https:// www.komen.org/breast-cancer/screening/when-to-screen/ average-risk-women/) and (https://www.touch4life.org/)

The decision to stop breast cancer screening depends on the health and condition of the woman and if she is expected to live at least 10 years. I typically am having this conversation with women who are relatively healthy and functioning well in the community and are most certainly likely to live at least another 10 years. I think that the most important factor in helping a woman decide about whether to continue breast cancer screening is to review with her whether the possible diagnostic testing that may be recommended is desired if the mammogram shows something abnormal (repeat testing, breast ultrasound, breast biopsy) and/or if breast cancer is diagnosed with a biopsy (surgery, radiation therapy, chemotherapy with oral pills or other modalities like intravenous medications). After having this discussion, some patients decide to NOT continue breast cancer screening because they feel whatever the outcome of the mammogram is, they would not want to proceed with further evaluation.

If the follow-up testing that will be needed based on the outcome of the test is not desired, you should consider not ordering the test. Unfortunately, once a test result is known, it is very difficult to return to the state of mind when the test result was not known. Knowing an undesirable test result or finding can cause a lot of anxiety when the next step that is now recommended for the results needs to be considered.

Patients are often very fixated on the ordering of tests instead of having the doctor take a detailed history of the symptoms or concerns in question to see if any testing is needed or warranted.

The discussion of the implications of ordering diagnostic imaging (X-rays, CT scans, MRI's, etc.) warrants the additional discussion of the fact that often things are found on diagnostic imaging that are unexpected and totally unrelated as to why the test was ordered. Many times, what is found on imaging is more serious than the problem that is being investigated by the test. This is good if the serious problem has a simple remedy, but often the problem found does not have an easy solution.

14

Dealing with Mediocrity and Incompetence from Others When Advocating for Yourself

*T*RYING TO GET WHAT YOU NEED FOR YOUR HEALTH WHEN you need it in this country's complicated healthcare system can be challenging.

This topic came up one day when talking to a patient about trying to navigate the healthcare system and her challenges in being an advocate for her health care needs. She was talking about the different challenges she has had over the years interfacing with medical professionals when her health needs were not managed as efficiently and precisely as they should have been. Fortunately, there were no glaring negligent issues that negatively affected her health because of this.

There are many things you can do to advocate for yourself to have your health care needs met:

- Sign up for the patient portal whenever your doctor or hospital system that you use has one.

- Use pharmacy online services when provided by your insurance company or local retail pharmacy where you can conveniently manage your pharmacy needs.
- Always follow up on prescription refill denials from the pharmacy by calling your insurance company to find out why payment was denied. You can assist your doctor and/or pharmacist with making decisions about your medication and medication alternatives and finding about the insurance company process to appeal the denial.
- Use mail order pharmacy benefits. Many find it very convenient to have 90 days supplies delivered to the home when feasible.
- Check with your insurance company about what vaccines are covered for you. Your doctor does not know your specific vaccine benefits.
- Check with your insurance company about what preventive health benefits are covered (preventive visit once a year, recommended screening blood tests and immunizations/vaccines).
- Check with your insurance company when diagnostic tests are ordered for you (x-rays, CT scans, MRI's etc.), if the radiology facility does not do this for you.
- Always follow up on insurance claim denials, including medication, doctor visits, hospital outpatient visit, inpatient stays, diagnostic testing, blood tests etc. Sometimes insurance claim denials are done in error and can be easily reversed. Often insurance companies have appeals processes that can lead to insurance claim denial reversals when you use the process to explain the medical need of the medical claim or request that has been denied. Often your doctor can assist you with this process

and it can be completed faster when you start the appeals process yourself with your insurance company.

- For seniors, contact your county senior services agency. Many agencies have case managers, social workers and referral resources that can help you advocate for you and help navigate health care challenges.

MAINTENANCE OF HEALTH

"Create your day and then create your life."
Prince

15

Simple Things You Can Do to Maintain Your Health

*A*S A PRIMARY CARE PHYSICIAN, I CARE FOR PATIENTS over many years, from the first visit until they move away, choose another physician, their insurance changes, they have not responded to telephone, patient portal message and/or postal letter outreach attempts, or until they transition at the end of their lives. Over time, I get to know them, hear their life stories, and meet their loved ones and caregivers. I have come to appreciate that the most significant practice that helps patients maintain health over time is how they structure their lives such that they feed their soul with activities and relationships to support mental capacity to attend to a healthy lifestyle and physical health and well-being.

People who have an overall positive sense of well-being are much better able to pay attention to making healthy choices in life that help prevent disease and attend to medical conditions and issues when and if they develop.

These are some concepts that I see people have (or avoid) that make their lives fulfilling and meaningful in the long run:

- Keep life simple.
- They don't under-appreciate the most seemingly inconsequential people who cross their path. Sometimes the best people to be in your life aren't the most sophisticated people. This makes me think of one of my patients who shared with me one visit that her greatest supporter is her adopted, behaviorally challenged son.
- Avoid and extricate themselves from toxic relationships and environments, including children, spouses, managers, co-workers.
- Get regular self-care treatments like massages, acupuncture, facials, engaging in relaxation techniques. You may have medical conditions or benefits where you can use medical insurance, health spending accounts (HSA) or flexible spending accounts (FSA) for these types of treatments.
- Take regular vacations, staycations and/or travel to visit friends and family.
- Participate in entertainment events and cultural events.
- Listen to music and read.
- Control exposure to media and environmental toxicities (including conversations that you have with people). Be mindful of the violence and profanity that you let in from visual, auditory, and written input into your brain. I have patients say all the time they limit being around negative people, including friends and family.

- Control exposure to commercial television, news, and social media. Make time to unplug from cell phones, computers, and radio.
- Take advantage of DVR's and television, radio apps and podcasts where you can plan to watch or listen to programs on demand, instead of adhering to scheduled broadcast times that interrupt your schedule. Then you can watch and listen faster because you can avoid commercials.
- Engage in whatever spiritual support works for you.
- Avoid nicotine, psychoactive drugs, unhealthy food, alcohol, being careful to not use these things to fill emotional voids within you.
- Have a low threshold to seek behavioral health counseling. Get psychological counseling to unpack unresolved psychological baggage and unresolved issues from childhood and earlier life. It is not a sign of weakness to get help managing feelings and emotions.
- Get at least 7 to 8 hours of sleep at night.
- Avoid working at night.
- Plan fertility.
- Regularly plan time alone.

16

The Importance of Following Up on Abnormal Test Results

I HAVE SEEN MANY NEW PATIENTS OVER THE YEARS WHO I find have abnormal test results when I review their previous medical records. It is often documented in the chart that the patient was told about the abnormal results. When asked about this, many patients confirm that they were aware of the abnormal results and did not follow up as recommended by their physician.

Here are a few significant abnormal results (and their implications in CAPS) that I often see in patients' medical records that were not followed up on and the diseases they could be increased risk for:

- Follow up colonoscopy for colon polyps removed with colonoscopy—COLON CANCER
- Abnormal Pap test results and/or HPV positive with Pap test—CERVICAL CANCER
- Follow up on abnormal mammogram findings—BREAST CANCER

- Follow up on elevated hemoglobin A1C (which means that you have pre-diabetes) —DIABETES, CHRONIC KIDNEY DISEASE, PERIPHERAL VASCULAR DISEASE, BLINDNESS
- Repeat testing for abnormal cholesterol tests (abnormal lipids) and they have not changed their eating habits to improve their cardiovascular risk-HEART ATTACK, STROKE, PERIPHERAL VASCULAR DISEASE
- Follow up on abnormal kidney function-CHRONIC KIDNEY DISEASE, END STAGE KIDNEY DISEASE, DIALYSIS
- Follow up on elevated blood pressure and uncontrolled high blood pressure (blood pressure consistently above 130/80) and/or stop taking high blood pressure medications—HEART ATTACK, STROKE, CHRONIC KIDNEY DISEASE, BLINDNESS.

ABNORMAL TEST OR FINDING	TEST THAT NEEDS TO BE DONE	POSSIBLE IMPLICATION
Colon polyps	Follow up Colonoscopy, follow up with the gastroenterologist	Colon cancer
Abnormal Pap test	Follow up Pap test, referral to GYN for further evaluation	Cervical cancer
Positive HPV test	Follow up Pap test with HPV co-testing, referral to GYN for further evaluation	Cervical cancer
Abnormal mammogram	Further breast imaging, consider seeing a breast specialist for further evaluation	Breast cancer
Abnormal hemoglobin A1C/ pre-diabetes	Repeat hemoglobin A1C blood test in 3 months	Diabetes, chronic kidney disease, artery/ circulation disease, blindness
Abnormal cholesterol test	Follow up cholesterol test in three months, advanced lipid testing https://www.healthline.com/health/cholesterol/advanced-cholesterol-test), coronary artery calcium score, https://www.healthline.com/health/heart-disease/coronary-calcium-score, consider seeing a cardiologist	Heart attack, stroke, artery/ circulation disease
Abnormal kidney function blood test	Repeat kidney blood test, consider seeing a kidney specialist	Chronic kidney disease, dialysis
Blood pressure too high	Regular blood pressure monitoring, regular doctor visits every 3-6 months	Chronic kidney disease, artery/ circulation disease, heart attack, heart failure, stroke

17

More on High Blood Pressure

HIGH BLOOD PRESSURE HAS BEEN CALLED "THE SILENT Killer" and can cause significant damage to internal organs (heart, brain, eyes, kidneys, circulation in legs and feet) over time without having any symptoms. Within my own practice, I have prescribed blood pressure medicine and then the patient stopped taking the medication and stopped checking their blood pressure. For example, I had a patient of a previous practice schedule a video visit to re-establish care with me in 2020. She told me we had last seen each other two years ago. She conveyed that previously I told her that her blood pressure was too high and that she should check her blood pressure at home. She reported she was not checking her blood pressure and didn't change her eating habits as we had discussed. She found me at my new practice and told me she was finally ready to follow up on her blood pressure.

She was asked to check her blood pressure on the day of the visit and told the medical assistant that her blood pressure was too high at 160/98 at home. (Optimal blood pressure is less than 120/80 and acceptable blood pressure is at least less than 130/80).

Additionally, I often review medical records from previous doctors and specialists for my new patients, interpreting past results. Countless times, I uncover significant issues in their medical records that the patient claims they were never informed about. When patients express frustration and concern when hearing the explanation of the abnormal test results from another doctor, I think to myself, "I am just the messenger." Often patients say, "No one ever told me this" or "Why didn't they tell me this?" My response is typically, "I don't know," but I let the patient know we have to proceed from here to evaluate the abnormal test result or finding. And at that point, I must address the abnormal results and initiate further evaluation that is needed.

Sometimes there has been a good amount of time between when the abnormal test results were available and the conversation that I am having with the patient. Sometimes this delay in evaluation leads to less-than-optimal outcomes.

With too much regularity, I have had patients admit they knowingly did not follow up on abnormal results because they were afraid of the implications. One patient in this situation explained to me why he did not follow up on his abnormal test result that he discussed with his previous doctor, which was a blood test that showed he was almost at the diabetes range. He said that he did not want to accept his test result. He also gave me his perspective about how to deliver information to patients regarding abnormal test results that the patient is not likely to want to hear; however, once there is agreement that a test is going to be ordered, it is expected that the patient will receive the results in a timely manner.

Resource for validated blood pressure machines:
https://www.validatebp.org/

How to check your blood pressure:
https://www.healthline.com/health/how-to-check-blood-pressure-by-hand

- You should have a blood pressure machine with an arm cuff (unless you are unable to use your upper arm to check your blood pressure)
- You should be quiet and at rest when you check your blood pressure

18

Outward Appearance Is Not What Ends Up Being Important

*H*AVING YOUR BODY LOOK THE WAY YOU WANT IT TO ON the outside can be misleading if you are not making choices about your health over time to optimize your internal bodily functions. Externally, we can see and then adorn and manipulate our hair, eyes, mouths, nails, skin, and clothes.

Instead, I recommend limiting the use of harmful chemicals with additives and parabens on the skin and hair. I recommend focusing on things that make you feel good and not what other people see.

It is important to not ignore dental hygiene and go to the eye doctor on a regular basis. Dental issues can cause and be a result of internal disease and eye exams can also reveal evidence of internal diseases.

Often, having insurance to get regular dental and eye exams are cost prohibitive for many people, even if you have some sort of medical/health insurance. You can often get free or low-cost dental exams at a student dental school if you can get to a university that has a dental school. In addition, you can contact your local health department for resources for low cost or free dental and eye care.

19

Ergonomics–Home Office and Work Office Furniture

WORKSTATION ERGONOMICS HAS BECOME INCREASINGLY important over the years as more people's work environment necessitates prolonged sitting/staring at a computer or screen while typing on a keyboard. All three of these functions (sitting, looking at a screen and typing) sets in motion a multitude of possible repetitive movement and strain injuries. Devices now include desktops, laptops, tablets, and smartphones.

Now that more people are working from home due to the pandemic in the United States in March 2020, I am seeing more patients with musculoskeletal complaints because many people do not have home workstations that are ergonomically correct. Working on the bed, couch, or kitchen table does not make for optimal ergonomic positioning without modifications that may need to be made as pictured in the diagrams on the following pages.

Prolonged sitting in front of or holding these devices causes common conditions, which can include:

- eye strain
- neck muscle strain
- back muscle strain
- shoulder pain
- finger pain
- numbness and tingling in the arms, elbows, wrists, hands, legs and/or feet originating from nerve irritation from muscle strain in the neck and back
- headaches

Proper workstation ergonomic information should be obtained from your employer, but I find that many employers offer no instruction on ergonomics and have inadequate desk and chair heights for the worker and inadequate keyboard and mouse/wrist supports and screen heights. Many employers purchase desks, chairs and workstations that are not adequately adjustable.

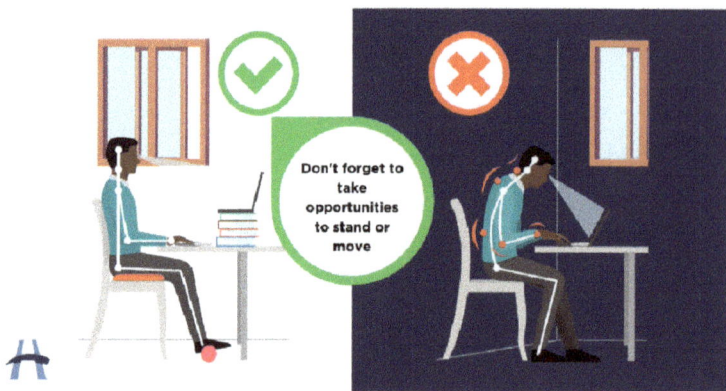

(https://www.hamiltonhealthsciences.ca/share/ergonomics -tips-for-working-remotely/)

Guide to an Ergonomic Workspace Setup

Screen position

Optimizing screen position **can help prevent neck pain and eye strain.**

Workspace surface

By avoiding overreaching and contact stress, this positioning **can minimize shoulder pain and wrist pain.**

Chair and foot support

Sitting in this position with adequate support **can help prevent to avoid back pain and shoulder pain.**

Knees should be level with hips.

The top of the monitor or laptop screen should be at eye level.

Screens should be about an arm's length away.

The external keyboard and mouse should be within close reach.

The table or desk should have enough room to rest forearms on the surface without raising shoulders or allowing soft tissue to dig into the surface's edge.

The chair should be at a height where you can rest your feet flat on the floor or an elevated surface, such as a stool.

Sources:

Mayo Clinic Staff. "Office Ergonomics: Your How-To Guide," Mayo Clinic, April 27, 2019.
https://www.mayoclinic.org/healthy-lifestyle/adult-health/in-depth/office-ergonomics/art-20046169

"The Ergonomic Journey—ErgoFit Consulting's Blog," ErgoFit Consulting.
https://ergofitconsulting.com/resources/ergofit-s-blog/960-what-they-didn-t-publish-from-our-business-insider-interview

(https://www.publichealthdegrees.org/resources/how-to-create-work-from-home-set-up/)

Ergonomics For Telecommuters

Ergonomics | Environmental & Occupational Health | FP&M | UW-Madison

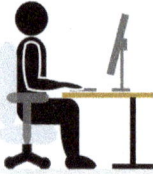

How To Set Up Your Workstation
To improve comfort, safety, and productivity anywhere

- Raise the top of your monitor to eye level or below
- Screen distance should be an arm's length away (18-30")
- Keep elbows at your sides and rest gently on armrests
- Maintain neutral wrists and forearms parallel to ground
- Rest feet flat on the floor with knees at or below hip level
  Leave 1" to 2" space between calves and the seat's edge

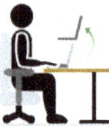

Using A Laptop?

- Raise your laptop to eye level
  Try a stand, box, or step stool
- And use a separate keyboard and mouse
- Or use a monitor and type on your laptop
  If you have a keyboard, mouse, and monitor, raise your laptop off to the side for dual monitors

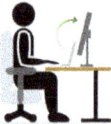

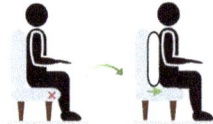

Sinking In Your Deep Couch?

- Use a pillow to shorten the seat
  A pillow or towel roll can also be used for lumbar support

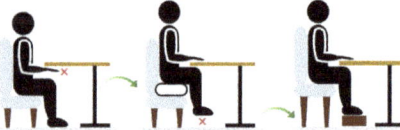

Work Surface Too High?

- Use a taller chair or raise your seat with a cushion
- Use a footrest or box to support your legs from dangling
- Type on a lower surface like a keyboard tray, lap desk, or side table

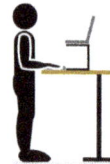

Prefer To Stand?

- Find a counter or tall surface
- Wear comfortable shoes
- Try standing on a kitchen mat

(https://www.uhs.wisc.edu/wp-content/uploads/2020/03/
Remote-Workspace-Ergonomics-3-18-20.pdf)

The theory of sitting or standing properly while working is to not sustain injury by straining your muscles.

- Focus on having proper head positioning which should be eye-level to your screen so you are not looking down or looking up.
- Focus on having good back support and good back posture, by not leaning backward or leaning forward.
- Limit prolonged looking down at your cell phone and limit prolonged texting on the cell phone.

More workplaces provide standing desks, but often patients are required to have a letter from their doctor documenting a medical need for a standing desk. A mechanical desk that allows both standing and sitting works for a lot of people.

- If your work involves driving or more vigorous activity, like lifting, reaching, climbing and bending and other activities, take care to get enough sleep such that fatigue does not lead to injury. Follow all recommended safety measures at your work site and use all recommended safety equipment. Take regular breaks to rest your muscles.

THE PAINLESS NATURE OF DIABETES, HIGH BLOOD PRESSURE, AND HIGH CHOLESTEROL

Don't think there are no crocodiles
just because the water's calm.
African Proverb

20

Diabetes

*D*IABETES IS STILL A SUBSTANTIAL CONTRIBUTOR TO people having heart disease, including heart attacks, peripheral vascular disease, toe, foot and leg amputations, blindness, and strokes. I believe the fact that diabetes itself does not cause pain makes diabetes very easy to ignore.

Diabetes is frequently diagnosed simply by doing a screening blood test (a blood test to screen for diabetes, which is recommended to be done every 3 years in all adults) without the patient having any symptoms. Currently diabetes is diagnosed when the hemoglobin A1C gets to 6.5% or a fasting glucose (blood sugar) of 126 or above or a non-fasting glucose 140 or above. We start considering taking medication for diabetes when the hemoglobin A1c gets to 7% to prevent the long-term complications of uncontrolled diabetes and the increased risk of cardiovascular disease, like heart attack and stroke. The hemoglobin A1c is simply how much sugar is attached to the red blood cells. This value is considered normal if it is 5.6% or less. (https://www.diabetes.org/a1c/diagnosis)

In some ways, the Hemoglobin A1C test is like a baseball player's season batting average. Both Hemoglobin A1C and the batting average tell you about a person's overall success.

The following can help you understand a hemoglobinA1C result:

- 4.0–5.6% Normal
- 5.7–6.4% Pre-Diabetes
- 6.5–6.9% Excellent control of Diabetes
- 7.0–7.9% Fair control of Diabetes—MEDICATION RECOMMENDED AT THIS LEVEL
- 8.0–8.9% Poor control of Diabetes
- 9.0% and above
- Very Poor control of Diabetes—CONSIDER INSULIN OR INJECTABLE DIABETES MEDICATIONS

HEMOGLOBIN A1C RESULT	MEANING
5-4–5.6%	NORMAL
5.7–6.4%	PRE-DIABETES
6.5–6.9%	EXCELLENT CONTROL OF DIABETES
7.0–7.9%	FAIR CONTROL OF DIABETES— MEDICATION RECOMMENDED AT THIS LEVEL
8.0–8.9%	POOR CONTROL OF DIABETES
9% AND ABOVE	VERY POOR CONTROL OF DIABETES— CONSIDER INSULIN AND/OR INJECTABLE DIABETES MEDICATIONS

Regrettably, it is easy for patients to ignore diabetes for years, and sometimes even decades, after diagnosis because it often doesn't cause symptoms or pain. In fact, kidney failure, stroke, heart attack, blindness, and limb amputation (all ultimately caused by the long-term complications of diabetes in small blood vessels) are hard for people to conceptualize happening to them in the future when no symptoms and/or pain are compelling the person to seek medical attention and/or make lifestyle changes (choosing healthier food, exercising). It is hard for a patient to look ahead to these types of issues when the small blood vessel disease that diabetes causes does not cause them any discomfort over the many years that it is going on undetected.

Ultimately, the problem with diabetes not causing direct symptoms is that the complications of diabetes that can cause chronic conditions that lead to progressive symptoms, the need to take multiple medications, the need to see physicians and specialists and the increased risk of chronic illness and death are present, but not being addressed.

Coronary artery disease (CAD-blocked arteries that give blood to the heart) can lead to chest pain and heart attacks. Medications are used to prevent worsening CAD and placing stents in the blocked heart arteries and doing surgery to bypass blocked arteries are possible treatments for CAD. Heart attacks can lead to heart rhythm problems, progressive congestive heart failure and uncontrolled heart failure. These conditions can cause leg swelling, weight gain, trouble breathing, fatigue and decreased energy, to name a few symptoms. The worse heart failure gets, the harder it is to control with medications. Depending on the cause of the heart failure, left ventricular assist devices (mechanical, implanted device to assist heart function), heart transplant and other newer interventions are possible treatments to end stage heart failure.

Of course, strokes can lead to the following complications, which can greatly alter your lifestyle through loss of independence, permanent disability and loss of mobility and death:

- Neurologic: weakness and paralysis of arms and legs, inability to speak and swallow, problems with thinking, visual problems, dementia and more
- Loss of eyesight, toe, foot, and leg amputations
- Kidney failure and end stage kidney disease, leading to dialysis also changes your lifestyle and can lead to other diseases and complications in other organs of the body (brain, heart especially) once the kidney failure reaches a certain level.

When patients are diagnosed with diabetes, they often struggle to accept the diagnosis because they don't have any symptoms and don't feel sick. Their typical second response is often expressing reluctance to take medication to treat diabetes. The primary treatment for Type 2 diabetes (typically adult onset, but more frequently occurring in the pediatric age group) is not always medication, but instead, the treatment is focused on improving eating habits, getting regular exercise and losing weight if the person is overweight. When I communicate this treatment plan, many patients are instantly relieved. Many patients do very well with controlling their diabetes without medication by eating a more plant-based diet, including consuming more vegetables, focusing on the lower sugar fruits, like berries and apples, and limiting protein to lean meats, like chicken, turkey and fish for meat. I do let people keep oatmeal and beans because of the beneficial effects from the fiber.

Often, depending on the glucose, the hemoglobin A1c level and the patient's other medical conditions, I recommend having the patient work on improving eating habits and getting regular exercise to see if the diabetes condition can be controlled without starting medication initially. I may recommend that they start checking glucose at home to monitor glucose in between visits with me. Many patients are able to do this by making significant changes in their eating habits. Often patients with newly diagnosed diabetes are still at the point where there is time to work on making lifestyle changes that can reverse diabetes. In addition, many patients who are already on medication when they start their care with me or even those who I've started on medication can improve their diabetes, such that the diabetes medication regimen can be de-escalated or eliminated with close monitoring with my supervision.

21

High Blood Pressure

IGH BLOOD PRESSURE, "THE SILENT KILLER", IS ANOTHER condition that causes no direct symptoms in many people but can be unsuspectingly causing organ damage for many years. Uncontrolled high blood pressure (hypertension) can cause the same constellation of symptoms and chronic disease risk leading to the final common pathway of vascular and end organ (brain, heart, eyes, kidneys, limbs) damage.

Blood pressure is the pressure of blood pushing against the walls of your arteries. Arteries carry blood from your heart to other parts of your body. Your blood pressure normally rises and falls throughout the day. An optimal blood pressure level is less than 120/80 mmHg, no matter your age, but blood pressure should consistently be less than 130/80 to prevent the long-term complications that can come from blood pressure above these goals. Blood pressure is measured using two numbers:

- The first number, called systolic blood pressure, measures the pressure in your arteries when your heart beats.

- The second number, called diastolic blood pressure, measures the pressure in your arteries when your heart rests between beats. (https://www.cdc.gov/high-blood-pressure/about/?CDC_AAref_Val=https://www.cdc.gov/blood-pressure/about.htm)

In general, it is currently recommended to start considering treating high blood pressure if the blood pressure is consistently 140/90 (130/80, if you have certain medical conditions like kidney disease, stroke or heart disease) or above. Just as with diabetes, blood pressure treatment should start with improving eating habits and getting regular exercise. Initial management of high blood pressure should include this lifestyle modification as well as daily home blood pressure blood pressure monitoring. And just as with diabetes, making the necessary lifestyle changes and checking the blood pressure daily at home can be done with close follow up and physician supervision before deciding about whether to start blood pressure lowering medication. (https://www.ncbi.nlm.nih.gov/pmc/articles/PMC4473614/)

I infrequently make decisions about blood pressure and whether blood pressure medication is needed by any one office blood pressure reading. I always encourage anyone who has an issue with blood pressure and/or is taking blood pressure medications to check their blood pressure daily because home blood pressure readings are more indicative of what a patient's blood pressure is than the blood pressure reading in the office. In addition, often blood pressure readings are elevated in the doctor's office and are much more controlled at home. I recommend that patients use the patient portal technology to send me their blood pressure readings, glucose readings and use the information on the patient portal to be better participants and their own health status. Alternatively, I recommend that patient's write down their blood pressure readings on paper daily and bring their blood pressure readings and blood pressure machine to their office visits, so that the blood pressure machine can be checked for correct arm cuff size, proper use and accuracy. I recommend checking blood pressure with an arm cuff (not a cuff that goes around the wrist or finger). We consider a blood pressure reading from the patient's machine to be accurate enough if the values are within 10 points (mmHg-millimeters of mercury, which is the unit of a blood pressure reading) of the value from the office blood pressure machine.

22

High Cholesterol

$\mathcal{H}$IGH CHOLESTEROL IS ANOTHER INSIDIOUS CONDITION that leads to vascular and end organ disease while causing no pain or other symptoms. It is recommended that all adults be screened for high cholesterol at least every 5 years and more often, depending on your health status and other medical conditions.

Broadly, cholesterol status is assessed by looking at specific components of cholesterol that are involved in causing vascular and organ problems. These components are:

- Total cholesterol
- HDL cholesterol
- LDL cholesterol
- Triglycerides

Under the age of 40, it is recommended that working on lifestyle modification, including making changes in eating habits and getting exercise, should be initiated to see if the cholesterol profile can be improved prior to age 40. Medication to improve the cholesterol should be considered beginning at age 40 if needed. If the LDL is above 190, then treatment should be considered, even if you are under age 40. Treatment should also be considered if the triglycerides are 600 or above.

In general:

- The total cholesterol should be less than 200.
- The LDL (bad cholesterol) should be less than 100. If you have diabetes, it should be less than 70 and if you have heart disease or diabetes.
- The triglycerides (fat in the blood) should be less than 200.
- The HDL (good cholesterol) should be more than 55.

Starting at age 40, assessment of cholesterol status involves doing a risk calculation based on additional factors other than your actual cholesterol numbers. An evaluation of cholesterol testing is INCOMPLETE without a risk assessment calculation. This is because the latest 2019 American Heart Association guidelines do not target specific cholesterol levels anymore, but rather base treatment of high cholesterol on calculated risk for atherosclerotic disease (heart attack, stroke and peripheral vascular disease). We try to estimate a person's risk of heart disease or stroke using a calculator designed by the American Heart Association and the American College of Cardiology. This risk calculator is based on age, ethnicity, blood pressure, diabetes status, smoking and cholesterol values (total cholesterol, HDL, LDL). (https://www.ahajournals.org/doi/10.1161/CIR.0000000000000678?url_ver=Z39.88-2003&rfr_id=ori:rid:crossref.org&rfr_dat=cr_pub%3dpubmed)

Based on cholesterol values and other cardiovascular risk factors, the predicted 10-year risk for atherosclerotic cardiovascular disease (ASCVD-https://www.healthline.com/health/stroke/stroke-screening) is a percentage that is then categorized to be in a low, borderline, intermediate or high-risk range. The use of cholesterol-lowering medication is felt to be beneficial when the calculated risk is in the intermediate to high-risk range. A calculation in the borderline risk range requires lifestyle modification and more frequent re-assessment.

This calculation risk factors include:

- Age (men are higher risk than women)
- Smoking status (smoking increases risk)
- Systolic (top number of the blood pressure reading) and diastolic (bottom number of the blood pressure reading) blood pressure (the higher the blood pressure above 120/80, the higher the risk)
- Diabetes (having diabetes infers higher risk)

Also included in the calculation is if the patient is black or white; being black assumes higher risk. I do not like this variable because race has no biological basis. These are social terms and are self-reported characteristics based on a phenotypic identification (how you look on the outside) instead of a genetic identification (what genes you have and what part of the world your genes are from). It would be more ideal if we had a more scientific variable that was clinically useful. Unfortunately, increased cardiovascular risk for patients defined as "black" has more to do with socioeconomic disparities rather than due to inherent characteristics due to the color of the patient's skin.

WHAT TESTS SHOULD YOU ASK YOUR DOCTOR TO ORDER FOR YOU?

FIRST, with respect to cholesterol and assessing your risk for heart disease:

- Lipid panel or lipid profile or cholesterol test at least every 5 years or more often all in adults, more often if you have abnormal results or you taking cholesterol lowering medication https://www.healthline.com/health/cholesterol-test

- If you are above age 40, your doctor should then do a risk assessment using the results of your lipid panel and other variables to assess your risk for heart attack and stroke. This is called RISK ASSESSMENT and there are various tests and tools that we use to do this to see who is at risk for heart attack and stroke, especially at age 40 and above, when your medical history, family history and lipid panel alone do not give a definitive answer. In general, checking a lipid panel without your doctor doing at least the risk assess scoring tool portion is not complete:

  - ASCVD (Atherosclerosclerotic Cardiovascular Disease) Risk Score https://www.healthline.com/health/stroke/stroke-screening

  - MESA (Multi-Ethnic Study of Atherosclerosis) score takes into account a Coronary Artery Calcium score (see below) and other variables that increase the risk of heart attack and stroke. It is another risk assessment tool.

    - https://internal.mesa-nhlbi.org/about/overview

  - Here are other tests that can give you more information about your risk of heart attack and stroke (other than your diet, your level of fitness/exercise, medical history and family history):

    - Coronary Artery Calcium Score https://www.healthline.com/health/heart-disease/coronary-calcium-score

- Lipoprotein A, Apoprotein A, Apoprotein B and other markers or Advanced Lipid Testing
- https://www.healthline.com/health/cholesterol/advanced-cholesterol-test
- https://www.youtube.com/watch?v=0zkLGawMtwc
- Carotid ultrasound (ultrasound of the arteries of the neck to see if you have blockages that give blood to the brain. If you do, you could have blockages in other arteries in your body, including that arteries that give blood to your heart) https://www.health line.com/health/carotid-duplex

GETTING TO YOUR WEIGHT LOSS GOAL

*Your food is supposed to be your medicine and
your medicine is supposed to be your food.*
African Proverb

23

Your Way is Not Working.... Try Something Different

T HIS IS SOMETHING THAT I OFTEN SAY TO PATIENTS WITH whom I am working to manage a medical issue. Often patients come to me with medical problems that have been going on for quite some time (months to years) and the person has come to me because the medical issue(s) are not controlled or resolved to the level of their satisfaction.

In general, when a new patient chooses me as their primary care physician, I start the evaluation by eliciting a complete story from them. I encourage the patient to recount their lifetime medical history, beginning in childhood, and share the health challenges they've faced throughout their life. I review medical records to assess for accuracy and to document the nuances to the information that I already have. Sometimes, this may take 2-3 visits if I have to wait for external medical records to fill in the blanks the patient is unaware of and/or has forgotten. Allowing the patient to narrate their life story from their perspective allows me to begin getting to know the patient and understand the full scope of what their life has been like up until our meeting. (https://www.cdc.gov/obesity/php/data-research/adult-obesity-facts.html?CDC_AAref_Val=https://www.cdc.gov/obesity/data/adult.html)

A common medical issue that I address with many patients on a daily basis is obesity. Many patients seek medical advice about how to lose weight. In the United States, obesity is an increasing medical problem that raises the risk of being diagnosed with and complicating many other serious and chronic medical conditions like COVID 19 infection, diabetes, heart disease, stroke, cancer and kidney problems.

This initial process is very effective for acquiring an understanding of the scope of experiences of a patient who has a goal of losing weight. I have the patient tell me what their previous weight evaluation has been and what methods of trying to lose weight have been tried in the past that have and have not worked:

- What specialists have been seen and what previous evaluations (blood work, imaging studies etc.) have been done
- What lifestyle changes, medications, therapies and/or treatments have been tried and what were the outcomes of these attempts
- Detailed review of eating patterns and food choices
- Review of how food intersects with their everyday life
- Review of their relationship and feelings/emotions about food and eating
- Review of mental health and psychological evaluations that impact making health food choices
- Review of medical history and medications that can impact weight and appetite

Patients often have tried to lose weight in the past and have been successful but have gained back unwanted weight. In these instances, reviewing and reconnecting with successful habits to achieve prior weight loss goals is all that may be needed.

In other cases, patients have tried lifestyle modification, eating habits, therapies, and treatments, but did not do it long enough or did not take a medication at a high enough dose to reach their goal. Often these types of modalities must be revisited and retried to maximize the desired weight loss response. Review of previous medical records to see what has been documented previously aids in this plan of action.

After the patient history of obesity and weight loss history and challenges have been reviewed, I make suggestions on a plan of action which some are frequently reluctant to try. Sometimes the obvious course of action to me has not been tried and has been suggested by other doctors that have evaluated the same weight loss goals with the patient. When I get to this hesitancy, I say to the person, "Because your way is not working, let's try my suggestions." This statement is often met with a pause in the patient's response and then fortunately a resolution to try something different. People are often frustrated with their lack of success with losing weight, and I strive to compose for them a realistic and sustainable approach to attaining their weight loss goals.

For the majority of people, the solution to achieving weight loss goals occurs by changing the relationship with food, changing food choices and having consistently planned daily eating. People feel a lot better about confronting their frustration and rising to the challenge of sticking to the plan of action once I have redirected them about planning to eat, planning food choices, eating regular meals, and keeping unhealthy foods out of their environment. Keys to success are:

- Avoiding cow's milk
- Avoiding egg yolks
- Avoiding cheeses
- Avoiding beef
- Focusing on eating lots of vegetables
- Focusing on eating low sugar fruits, if fruit is to be consumed at all (lemons, limes, strawberries, raspberries, blackberries, kiwi, avocado)
- Preferentially choosing baked chicken, turkey and fish (not shellfish), if meat is to be consumed
- Limiting starches, sugar and sweetened beverages (beans/legumes and oatmeal are generally OK)
- Eating food cooked at home (avoiding food from restaurants)

Patients are encouraged when I remind them how much more economical it is to focus on eating food cooked at home instead of eating out as much.

A further matter that has to be addressed is making the patient aware that everyone in their life environment (home and work) has to be engaged in not sabotaging the patient's progress by bringing unhealthy foods into their environment. I encourage the patient to involve their entire household in making sure that unhealthy foods are removed from the home (or at least hidden from the patient) and not brought back into the home. In addition, grocery shopping and healthy food preparation at home goes more smoothly if everyone in the home is committed to eating healthier to support the person with their weight loss and lifestyle modification efforts. It is exhausting and time consuming to make separate meals for everyone's various food desires in the household. This becomes particularly challenging if a person lives with other adults who ultimately are NOT going to support and even join the patient in the weight loss journey. Commonly, people have to go it alone at home in this process, but this makes it more difficult to reach weight loss targets, if the ability of the patient to avoid food contraband in their environment is compromised on a daily basis

There are many medical conditions that are improved by aggressively encouraging people to develop a more plant-based focus to eating:

- Diabetes
- High blood pressure
- High cholesterol
- Heart disease
- Kidney disease
- Stroke
- Circulation problems in the legs
- Inflammatory, connective tissue and autoimmune disorders, including lupus, rheumatoid arthritis, fibromyalgia, and other related conditions
- Arthritis
- Anxiety and depression

In addition, I commonly recommend chiropractor, acupuncture, and naturopathic practitioner (alternative medicine, complementary medicine, integrative medicine) evaluations, which all can help people focus on a holistic approach to their lifestyle modification changes, especially when/if chronic illnesses are present. Many people have never been introduced to these types of evaluations and I encourage people to try them before deciding that they will not be effective.

To help move the patient past their inertia, I explore any underlying reasons for their resistance to following previous recommendations or their current reluctance to try the suggestions

I am making. Often a person's reluctance to undertake a new way of thinking and embarking on a new plan of action can be transformed by having a person be honest with themselves about their reservations and barriers to moving forward with doing something different. I have found that frequently, reluctance in this process has nothing to do with what is being recommended, but is often related to fear of making changes, fear of exiting the comfort zone to think in a different way and fear of failing in their attempt at losing weight again. Other obstacles include listening to ill-advice from others and listening to those who have had a negative outcome from a particular treatment. A negative outcome with a therapeutic process in one person does not mean that it will not work in someone else. Individuals are not the same and a therapy or lifestyle modification for one person cannot be compared to another individual. I expressed to them that they should consider trying something different to see if they can feel better and they won't know if a particular treatment plan will not work unless they try it.

The overarching goal when met with patient resistance in this evaluation is to impress upon them that they have no chance of feeling better, improving, and getting to weight loss and chronic disease management goals unless they are willing to retry things to get the maximum effect or try methods they have not tried before.

24

Change Your Relationship with Food OR Food Is Not Your Friend

HEN OBESITY, MORBID OBESITY, JOINT PAIN (LOW BACK pain, hip pain, knee pain, ankle pain, foot pain), cardiovascular risk diseases (diabetes, pre-diabetes, high blood pressure, high cholesterol), heart attacks, strokes, worsening kidney failure, being on dialysis, vascular disease in the legs and feet, amputations of the lower extremities are affecting patients in varying degrees, I ultimately have to tell patients that food is not their friend anymore. Many people eat out of boredom, engage in emotional eating, and eat for taste and pleasure, instead of eating for just for health and nutrition's sake. However, when these disease types set in and start to escalate, you cannot continue to have the same relationship with food anymore. At this point, I recommend the patient explore and expand other aspects of their life to find pleasure other than eating.

The other problem is that eating and food are a big part of many of our social events and gatherings, even virtual events since

March 2020. I advise that people eat before participating in social events, so they can eat small amounts during the event, such that they do not feel like they are missing out on anything and so others will not comment on what they are and are not eating.

The bottom line is when you are dealing with these kinds of health conditions and medical issues, you must change what you habitually associate with food and eating and transform the place that food has in your life. I recommend that people remove all the junk food, unhealthy snacks and high sugar and high fat foods out of the house and only bring in healthy foods. With this practice, if you want to eat something unhealthy on occasion, you can go out and get it, eat a serving and be done with it and not have the food in the home, such that it is not in your presence, threatening to sabotage the efforts to eat healthier.

Once the atherosclerotic disease (blockages in arteries), end organ damage (organ damage from blocked arteries) and microvascular disease (blockages in the small arteries that give blood to organs) ball starts rolling down the hill, it is hard to reverse. When these diseases have started, making small, incremental changes and "eating everything in moderation" as many of my patients want to do, is not enough.

Here are tips that I review with patients to help them aggressively begin healing and halt disease progression:

- Plan to eat like you plan everything else that you do every day; you should know what you are going to eat every day when you wake up.
- Change your relationship with food.
- Eat for nutrition's sake, not for boredom or emotional eating.
- Find other pleasures in life besides eating.

- Eat before you go out for dinner, parties, and gatherings, especially between Thanksgiving Day and New Year's Day.
- Keep healthy snacks in the home and remove ice cream and junk food from the home.
- Take healthy snacks with you when you leave home to avoid drive-thru, fast food and take out restaurant food while at work, doing errands and traveling to and from work.
- Carry healthy snacks in a portable cooler bag with cold packs, if needed, to keep healthy perishable snacks cool, especially in the summer.
- Take water with you when leaving the home to make sure that water intake throughout the day is sufficient.
- Make sure that you consciously consider why you are eating, every time that you eat.
- Eat something small at regular intervals of every 3-4 hours, because it is time to eat, whether you are hungry or not, so avoid eating to chase hunger.
- Focus on adding movement to daily activities including, walking, and cycling outside or on exercise equipment, doing yard work, gardening, water exercises, etc.
- Focusing on changing food choices is more impactful than focusing on vigorous exercise. You can't exercise away a bad diet.
- Choose fresh foods that are as close to their natural state as possible, avoiding processed foods and processed meats (bacon, sausage, ham, deli meats, cold cuts, hot dogs), focusing on eating vegetables (fresh or frozen, not pre-seasoned) and fruits (fresh and frozen, no added sugar).
- Limit milk and cheese from a cow.
- Limit food from packages and cans.

- Write down what you eat and what time you eat to hold yourself accountable to what you are consuming. There are many apps that serve this purpose.
- Read food labels to limit sugar and sodium in food that you eat.
- Avoid sweetened cereals.
- Limit alcohol and beer intake.
- Avoid sugar, processed sugar foods and sweetened beverages, including fruit juices.
- Sleep at least 6-8 hours every 24 hours.
- Obesity and accompanying high blood pressure, high cholesterol and diabetes is significantly improved by cutting down and even eliminating starches (bread, rice, pasta white potatoes).
- Focus on eating lower sugar fruits (lemons, limes, strawberries, raspberries, blackberries, kiwi, avocado).
- If you want something "unhealthy" on occasion, you can go out of your home and get one serving of it rather than keeping it in the home. Understand that this does not mean doing this weekly or even monthly for some foods.

A WORD ABOUT INTERMITTENT FASTING

I am not a huge fan of intermittent fasting. Intermittent fasting does not work for everyone who tries to do it to lose weight and it is not a sustainable way to eat and live. Intermittent fasting focuses on eating within a certain time window, which does not fit everyone's lifestyle. In order to lose weight, you have to eat a certain amount to avoid putting your body in starvation mode (you hold onto everything that you eat and WILL NOT lose weight). Many people set an eating window for themselves but do not eat enough during that window to lose weight. It also makes many people think about eating too much, which makes it harder to have controlled eating.

You should be giving your body and brain nutrients when you are using them, which begins when you wake up. Not eating until mid-morning is not physiologic in the sense that your body is functioning, but you have not given it any nourishment to the cells of your body to function.

Here are some things to consider before trying intermittent fasting:

- Everyone does intermittent fasting…you are fasting while you are asleep!
- Discuss intermittent fasting with your doctor to see if it is appropriate for you.
- Most people have long days and your brain needs nutrition while you are awake. Intermittent fasting can mean that you are not eating while you still need to be awake (and not drowsy) and still need nutrition to function.
- Thinking about when you are going to eat next and thinking about getting food in by a certain time may not be a sustainable lifestyle. Being hungry is no way to live.
- Intermittent fasting can result in headaches and not feeling well.
- https://www.healthline.com/nutrition/intermittent-fasting-side-effects

25

Kick the Sandwich Habit

W HEN YOU ARE TRYING TO LOSE WEIGHT, REVERSE PRE-
diabetes and/or control diabetes, eating sandwiches can
be a compact source of too much starch, fat, and salt. In addition to the bread of a sandwich, what we put inside sandwiches
can also be a source of salt and fat in the form of processed meats
(deli meats/cold cuts, hot dogs, bacon, sausage), red meat (beef
burgers), condiments (mayonnaise and spreads), and sugar in
the form of peanut butter with added sugar and jelly/jams.

A common discussion I have with patients is how to control
the food in their home environment when other people that they
live with are not on their same journey to make healthier food
choices. I encourage patients to take the handouts that I have reviewed and given to them during our visits and sit down with
their family members to see if they can get them engaged in having the entire family commit to eating healthier. This can mean
that everyone in the home can be held accountable for not bringing food "contraband" into the house. One is less likely to eat
unhealthy food, if it is not readily available and healthy alternatives are available and being cooked instead.

HEALTHY FOOD CHOICES

MEATS/FISH

- Choose skinless, lean meats (chicken, turkey, fresh or frozen fish, canned fish packed in water). Meats and fish should be broiled or baked.

EGGS

- Egg substitutes and egg whites (use freely). Egg yolks (limit to 2-3 egg yolks per week).

FRUITS

- Eat 1-2 servings of fresh, low sugar fruit (apples, lemons, limes, strawberries, raspberries, blackberries, kiwi, avocado) per day (1 serving = 1/2 cup), if you are eating fruit in your diet. Frozen or canned fruit with NO sugar or syrup added may be used.

VEGETABLES

- Most vegetables are not limited (see Foods to Avoid below). At least 2 servings daily of vegetables are recommended (1 serving = 1 cup raw or ½ cup cooked). It is preferable to eat raw or steamed vegetables, but they may be lightly boiled as well. Heavily boiled vegetables take away the nutrients and fiber of the vegetable.

BEANS

- Dried peas or beans (1 serving = 1/2 cup) may be used as a bread substitute. Canned beans can be used if needed, but they should be drained and rinsed.

NUTS

- Unsalted almonds, walnuts, peanuts, pumpkin, sesame, or sunflower seeds can be eaten in small amounts daily.

MILK PRODUCTS

- Choose plant-based milk options: soy milk, rice milk, almond milk, cashew milk.

FATS/OILS

- Current recommendations are to use extra virgin or virgin olive oil (not heated past 350 degrees) and avocado oil most often. Soft (not stick) unsalted margarine, vegetable oils that are high in polyunsaturated fats (PUFA's), such as safflower, sunflower, soybean, corn, cottonseed, are no longer recommended as the main source of unsaturated fat. PUFAs, especially Omega 6 fatty acids, if consumed often enough, can produce pro-inflammatory (promoting inflammations) factors in the body. People can get high levels of these harmful factors in the body through frequent fried food intake.
- https://www.healthline.com/nutrition/optimize-omega-6-omega-3-ratio#TOC_TITLE_HDR_5

DESSERTS/SNACKS

- Sugar free gelatin and pudding, fresh fruit are good options for desserts.

BEVERAGES

- Water, black coffee, plain or herbal teas and sugar free soft drinks are good beverage options.

MISCELLANEOUS
- You may use the following freely: vinegar, no sodium spices, seasonings and herbs; non-fat and no or low sodium broths, mustard, low sodium Worcestershire sauce, low sodium soy sauce.

FOODS TO AVOID BY CATEGORY

MEATS/FISH
- Beef, processed pork, bacon, sausage, ham, fatty fowl (duck, goose), skin and fat of turkey and chicken, processed meats, luncheon meats (deli meats like salami, bologna), hot dogs, frankfurters and fast-food hamburgers (they are loaded with fat); organ meats (kidneys, liver); canned fish packed in oil. Even the turkey versions of processed meats and deli meats are just as harmful as the beef and pork versions.

EGGS
- Limit egg yolks to 2-3 per week.

FRUITS
- Coconuts (rich in saturated fat). Limit higher sugar fruits (pears, melons, bananas, grapes, cherries, pineapples, mango, peaches, nectarines and citrus fruits) if you are trying to lose weight and/or if you are trying to control your blood glucose for diabetes. Smaller portions of avocado should be eaten due to its high fat content.

VEGETABLES

- Starchy vegetables (potatoes, corn, peas) may be eaten if they are substitutes for a serving of bread or cereal.

BEANS

- Commercial baked beans with sugar and/or pork added.

NUTS

- Avoid salted nuts.

BREADS/GRAINS

- For weight loss and diabetes purposes, avoiding starches (bread, rice, pasta and white potatoes), including cereal (except for oatmeal) goes a long way to getting you to your health goals. Avoid baked goods with shortening and/or sugar, commercial mixes with dried eggs and whole milk, sweet rolls, doughnuts, pastries, toaster goods, sandwiches, buns, rolls, crackers, biscuits, toast, French toast, pancakes, waffles, English muffins and sweetened packaged cereals.

MILK PRODUCTS

- Cow milk and cow milk packaged goods, cream, ice cream, sweetened puddings, full fat and sugar yogurt, cheeses, non-dairy cream substitutes.

FATS/OILS

- Butter, lard, animal fats, bacon drippings, gravies, cream sauces, as well as palm and coconut oils. All these are high in saturated fats. Examine labels on cholesterol free products for hydrogenated fats. (These are oils that have been hardened into solids and in the process have become saturated.)

DESSERTS/SNACKS
- Fried snack foods like potato chips, pretzels, chocolate, candy, jams, jellies, syrups, sweetened puddings, ice cream, ice milk, sherbets, hydrogenated peanut butter.

BEVERAGES
- Fruit juices and sweetened soft drinks, cocoa made with whole milk and/or sugar. Limit alcohol.

HEALTHY EATING AND EXERCISE TIPS

Maintaining a lifestyle that keeps your heart healthy is one of the most important things that you can do. Illnesses caused by cardiovascular diseases (diseases of the heart and the blood vessels that give blood to the various organs of the body) are the leading cause of illness and death in this country. Heart disease causes more deaths than cancers in the United States. The prevention of various conditions like heart attack, stroke, high blood pressure, diabetes and kidney disease can be initiated by consistent lifestyle changes. (https://www.cdc.gov/nchs/fastats/leading-causes-of-death.htm)

- Regular exercise is the key to maintaining a healthy heart. Adequate exercise is any activity where you can get your heart rate up for at least 30 minutes, 3-5 times per week. Activities like walking and water aerobics are excellent ways to exercise.
- Healthy eating habits can go a long way to prevent cardiovascular disease.
- Start every day with breakfast (not necessarily breakfast food). This habit can help give you energy throughout

the day and prevent the feelings of hunger that limit your ability to choose healthy foods later in the day.

- Eat 3-6 small meals per day. A meal can be as small as a piece of fruit or a small salad. Healthy snacks prevent hunger and help you sustain energy for the day.
- Drink at least 8 glasses of water per day.
- Eat fresh, lean meats, like chicken, turkey, and fish. Limit more fatty meats, like beef and duck. You should limit all salt cured meats, like ham, cold cuts, bologna and hot dogs, bacon, and sausage.
- Limit your intake of salt (sodium). High sodium intake can increase blood pressure. High blood pressure damages blood vessels and organs. Sodium intake can be decreased by avoiding canned foods and processed boxed and microwaveable food products.
- Avoid all fried foods and fast foods. Low-fat food choices are now more available on many restaurant menus. Foods high in fat and cholesterol (like fried foods), high-fat snacks (like chips, candy bars, pastries, cakes, pies, and cheese) can raise your cholesterol levels and cause blockages in important arteries in the body. Arteries giving blood to the heart, brain, eyes, legs, and kidney need to be open for these organs to work properly.
- Eat no more than 3 eggs per week and limit the use of regular butter to decrease the high cholesterol content in your meals. Try low-fat versions of the foods you like. Drinking reduced fat milk and/or skim milk is best. Try rice, almond, cashew, or soy versions of the milk products that you like.
- Avoid all processed sugar foods and sweets, like pastries, baked goods, ice cream, candy and sweetened/bottled beverages.

- Drink water or sugar-free flavored water for your beverages.
- Eat lots of vegetables. Eat more fresh fruit instead of bottled juices and pop or soda.
- Cut down on all bread, rice, pasta, and white potatoes.

By eating healthier and doing regular exercise, you can be more successful at getting rid of excess pounds. Normal weight loss is just 4-5 pounds per month. The slow, steady shedding of excess weight by using healthy eating and exercise is more likely to be permanent than using fad diets. Be patient and consistent with your weight loss routine.

MAKING GOOD FOOD CHOICES WHEN EATING OUT

HOW TO MAKE A HEALTHY CHOICE AT RESTAURANTS

Restaurant food is inherently high in salt. If you are going to eat out, focus on ordering salads with the dressing on the side and avoid fried foods and foods with sauces and gravy on top.

Avoid salad bars, hot food bars and pre-prepared food venues, unless you are going to eat the fresh fruit and vegetables. (Beware, a lot of food put into salad bars comes out of a can, box or plastic pre-prepared package which is high in salt).

Many restaurants have healthy options and calorie content designated on the menu. Focus on these healthier food options.

- Avoid sweetened beverages, juices, and alcohol. Instead, order water with lemon or sugar free choices as your beverage.

- Drink water frequently during the meal to achieve the sensation of feeling full faster.
- Many restaurant portions are much larger than you need or even want to eat. When your food comes to you, place half of it in a take home box.
- Focus on ordering choices with fruits and vegetables as the predominant ingredients.
- If you are going to eat meat, avoid beef and focus on choices with chicken, turkey and fish that are baked, roasted or grilled, and not fried.
- Avoid processed meats, like deli meats, bacon, ham and sausage, including the turkey versions of these foods. While processed turkey is a better option than bacon, ham, and sausage, because the turkey is processed in the same manner, it can be just as harmful to your body. It may contain just as much or nearly as much salt and fat.
- Avoid salty snacks and sugary foods, pastries, candy and baked goods.
- Avoid choices rich with butter and rich sauces (these are high in fat).
- Minimize starchy foods like bread, rice, pasta and white potatoes. Substitute the starch in a meal for another vegetable. If you are going to eat starches, whole wheat or whole grain bread and pasta are better choices.
- Ask the server not to bring bread to the table while you are waiting for your meal.
- Do not add salt to your food. Only add salt to your food on your plate after you have tasted your food-use salt very sparingly, if at all.
- Avoid choices made with eggs and cheese.

- When planning to go out to eat or to an event, eat a small healthy snack before you go. Eat a snack high in protein such as tuna fish, seasoned by adding a little spicy brown mustard or low sodium salsa and eat with slices of your favorite vegetable like cucumbers or red bell pepper. You will eat less and be able to make healthier choices because you are not as hungry when you are ordering your meal.

Here are examples of health snacks with 200 calories or less:

1. One tablespoon peanut butter spread on slices of a medium apple
2. One cup tomato soup with five whole-grain crackers
3. Three cups air-popped popcorn sprinkled with three tablespoons grated parmesan cheese
4. Tri-color veggie snack: 6 baby carrots, 10 sugar snap peas (or green pepper strips), 6 cherry tomatoes and 2 tablespoons light dressing for dipping
5. Quick salad: 2 cups mixed greens with ½ cup sliced strawberries, 1 tablespoon sliced almonds and 1-2 tablespoons reduced-fat dressing
6. Red bell pepper slices with ⅓ cup guacamole
7. One cup cucumber slices with 2 tablespoons hummus
8. Chia pudding (made with chia seeds, non-dairy milk, ½ cup berries, your favorite extract for flavor
9. Seasoned roasted baby carrots
10. A boiled egg with ¼ sliced avocado and ¼ cup pistachios

DIABETES AND WEIGHT LOSS EATING HABITS

Some or all of these tips have been mentioned earlier, but I wanted to really focus on diabetes food management in particular.

- Eat within an hour of waking up every day.
- Every morning, you should know what you are going to eat and when you are going to eat it. You must plan to eat. If you do not plan to eat, you will eat foods that you should not be eating.
- It is ideal to eat small amounts of healthy foods at least 4-6 times a day.
- Food/snack prep and pack up your healthy snacks, so you can take your healthy snacks with you instead of eating out during the day.
- You should be eating something every 3-4 hours. You do not have to wait until you are hungry to eat something every 3-4 hours. In fact, going too long between meals will cause overeating.
- Focus on eating lots of vegetables and proteins like beans, chicken, turkey and fish that are baked and broiled, and not fried.
- Stick to eating low sugar fruits, like berries and apples. Avoid high sugar foods like melons, bananas, grapes, cherries, pineapples and citrus fruits. If you eat a high sugar fruit, eat a small amount (1 cup of watermelon, 1 orange, 8-10 grapes, 8-10 cherries). That is all of the fruit you should eat that day.
- Drink only unsweetened beverages. Avoid all juices, sodas, and all alcohol.

- Avoid eating bread, rice, pasta, white potatoes, including sandwiches, buns, rolls, crackers, toast, biscuits, cornbread, French toast, waffles, pancakes, bagels, and English muffins. Avoid eating cereals, except for oatmeal, that is not sweetened with sugar. Sweet potatoes are acceptable to eat if they are not eaten with added butter and sugar.
- Avoid butter, milk, and cheese from a cow. Try non-cow products like soy milk, rice milk, cashew milk and almond milk products that are unsweetened.
- Eat no more than 3 egg yolks per week. Focus on eating just egg whites instead.
- Stop eating processed sugar and baked sweets, including cakes, cookies, pies, donuts and avoid ice cream, sherbet, candy.
- Avoid packaged and processed foods in cans, boxes and plastic containers.
- Avoiding eating out at restaurants and fast-food establishments. Most of what you eat should be food that you prepared for yourself at home.

FLAVORING FOODS WITHOUT SALT

Focusing on eating food that is low in salt is a healthier way to eat overall. In general, food cooked at home is much lower in salt content than food purchased out of the home. Salt can raise blood pressure and a high salt diet can mean the difference between needing to take daily blood pressure medication or not.

Here are a few tips to lower the salt content of what you are eating on a regular basis:

- Avoid canned food, pre-packaged meals, processed foods and food in boxes and plastic containers.

- Avoid cheese. Cheese is high in salt.
- There are many ways to lower your sodium intake without sacrificing flavor. You might try herbs, spices, and seasoning blends when cooking. Here is a list of some options for adding taste and zest to your food without using extra salt.

Create your favorite flavors using herbs and spices:

- Bay leaf
- Cumin
- Curry
- Dill
- Dry mustard
- Green pepper
- Lemon juice
- Marjoram
- Onion
- Paprika
- Parsley
- Savory
- Basil
- Cloves
- Horseradish
- Nutmeg
- Pepper
- Rosemary
- Sage
- Thyme
- Oregano
- Poultry seasoning
- Saffron
- Sage
- Tarragon
- Thyme
- Allspice
- Cinnamon
- Garlic
- Ginger
- Poppy seed
- Celery seed

Some people find it easier to focus not on what they shouldn't eat, but instead, what they should eat. Here is a different way to look at healthy eating from a vantage point of weight loss and controlling blood glucose:

HEALTHY FOOD CHOICES

LOWER SUGAR FRESH FRUITS—
UNSWEETENED, NO ADDED SUGAR

- Apples
- Blueberries
- Mixed berries
- Raspberries
- Strawberries
- Blackberries

ALL NON-STARCHY VEGETABLES—
HERE ARE EXAMPLES:

- Tomatoes
- Cherry tomatoes
- Cucumber
- Roma tomatoes
- Asparagus
- Bell peppers
- Red peppers
- Yellow peppers
- Orange peppers
- Broccoli
- Brussels sprouts
- Cabbage
- Carrots
- Cauliflower
- Green beans
- Kale
- Lettuce
- Mixed greens
- Arugula
- Collard greens
- Mustard greens
- Mushrooms
- Onions
- Green onions
- Scallions
- Spaghetti squash
- Acorn squash
- Butternut squash
- Spinach
- Sweet potatoes
- Zucchini

SNACKS

- Unsweetened applesauce

NON-DAIRY BEVERAGE OPTIONS—
CHOOSE THE UNSWEETENED OPTIONS

- Soy milk
- Rice milk
- Cashew milk
- Almond milk

NON-FAT DAIRY OPTIONS

- Nonfat skim milk
- Nonfat cream cheese spread
- Nonfat, low-sodium, cottage cheese
- Nonfat Greek yogurt
- Nonfat half-and-half
- Nonfat sour cream
- Nonfat, low-calorie yogurt

SOUPS—MUST BE LOW-SODIUM
OR UNSALTED, SOUP IS ALWAYS
HEALTHIER WHEN IT IS HOMEMADE

- Vegetable and chicken broth
- Butternut squash soup
- Cabbage soup
- Chicken noodle soup
- Miso soup
- Spinach soup
- Tomato and lentil soup
- Vegetable barley soup

PROTEIN—EGGS, FISH AND MEAT

- Egg whites
- Any beans (dried beans are better than canned beans, canned beans should be rinsed): Black beans, black eyed peas, navy beans, red beans, lentils, kidney beans etc.
- Tofu
- Fish filets, baked, broiled, grilled, not fried-haddock, cod, halibut, tuna, tilapia, salmon etc.
- Baked chicken
- Baked turkey
- Ground turkey
- Ground chicken
- Canned tuna and water, not oil

CONDIMENTS-LOW-SODIUM AND LOW SUGAR PREPARATIONS ARE PREFERRED

- Buffalo sauce
- Hot sauces
- Lemon juice
- Lime juice
- Salsa
- Tomato sauce
- Tomato paste
- Vinegars (red wine vinegar, white vinegar) apple cider vinegar, rice vinegar, Balsamic vinegar)
- Mustard
- Ketchup

BEVERAGES

- Water
- Coffee
- Tea
- Low-sodium vegetable juice

READING FOOD LABELS

- https://www.fda.gov/food/nutrition-facts-label/how-understand-and-use-nutrition-facts-label
- https://www.heart.org/en/healthy-living/healthy-eating/eat-smart/nutrition-basics/understanding-food-nutrition-labels
- https://www.nia.nih.gov/health/how-read-food-and-beverage-labels
- https://www.healthline.com/nutrition/how-to-read-food-labels

26

The Work Break Room Will Sabotage You (The Break Room Will Kill You)

FOR THOSE THAT ARE GOING BACK TO WORK OUTSIDE OF the home now that indoor assembling and physical distancing restrictions are being reduced (or not adhered to), the break room at work again rears its evil head as a relentless source of high fat, high sugar, high cholesterol, high starch food and snacks and sweetened beverages.

Sharing food between co-workers and colleagues is a form of socialization in the workplace that is tempting and hard to avoid. Co-worker encouragement and peer pressure to consume food and beverages that have been brought to work to share for specific occasions, events, and even for no particular purpose, is an enticement that is difficult to escape. Potluck events in the workplace are difficult to avoid, especially if co-workers have a personal response to your polite declination to partake in the food that has been prepared.

I offer one talking point to patients so they can graciously avoid the work potluck: "My doctor told me that I cannot eat that."

My patients consistently come back to tell me that this statement facilitates them avoiding food they do not want to eat and avoiding hurt feelings from their co-workers.

Eating even when you are not hungry is a means that many people use to pass time while doing routine tasks at work.

To avoid the break room trap, I encourage patients to:

- Avoid the break room at all costs.
- Bring healthy meals, snacks, and beverages to work to avoid uncontrolled snacking on unhealthy foods and beverages.
- Briefly and nonchalantly inform coworkers of your desire to eat healthier and request that they not bring and offer food and beverages to your workstation.
- Bring healthy snacks to meetings to avoid the high fat and high sugar foods that are frequently available at workplace and business meetings.

In addition, I recommend avoiding the habit of having high sugar, high salt and high fat foods and beverages stored at your own workstation. This is also a frequent source of food and beverages that you should be trying to avoid that will be readily available for consumption if you keep them close to you.

27

Avoid Sugar and Processed Foods

THE SWITCH TO GET SUGAR AND PROCESSED FOODS OUT OF the environment is a challenge for many who are trying to make a nutritional shift in life. It is obvious that candy, jams, jellies, table sugar, honey and syrups, cakes, cookies, pies, doughnuts, ice cream, fruit juices, sodas and alcohol have to be significantly eliminated. Condiments, salad dressings, sauces and spreads in jars are notoriously high in sugar. As previously stated, the best way to avoid unhealthy ingredients is to focus on eating fresh foods and avoid foods that are in cans, boxes and packages. Often these preparations are high in salt (sodium) and sugar. Finding hidden sugar requires knowing the ingredients found on food labels that are sugar. Unfortunately, sugar is almost ubiquitous in most processed and prepared foods.

Here are the words, by category, to look for on food labels that still mean sugar:

CANE SUGAR

- Blackstrap molasses
- Brown sugar
- Cane juice/sugar/extract
- Caster sugar
- Coffee sugar crystals
- Demerara sugar
- Golden syrup
- Icing sugar
- Invert sugar
- Molasses
- Panela
- Rapadura
- Raw sugar
- Treacle
- Turbinado sugar
- White sugar

FRUIT

- Date sugar/syrup
- Fruit juice concentrate
- Fruit juice/sugar
- Grape sugar/syrup

BEET

- Beet sugar

CORN

- Corn syrup/sugar
- Glucose syrup
- High fructose corn syrup

ALTERNATIVE SWEETENERS

- Agave
- Barley malt syrup
- Brown rice syrup
- Coconut sugar
- Date sugar
- Honey Malt extract
- Maple syrup
- Palm sugar
- Rice malt syrup

CHEMICAL NAMES

- Glucose
- Dextrose (another name for glucose)

- Fructose (fruit sugar)
- Lactose (milk sugar)
- Maltose (malt sugar)
- Sucrose

(https://www.sugarnutritionresource.org/the-basics/sugars-on-food-labels)

THE MANY NAMES FOR SUGAR (LIST)

(https://sugarscience.ucsf.edu/hidden-in-plain-sight/#.YOt L8nlKiUk)

- Agave nectar
- Barbados sugar
- Barley malt
- Barley malt syrup
- Beet sugar
- Brown sugar
- Buttered syrup
- Cane juice
- Cane juice crystals
- Cane sugar
- Caramel
- Carob syrup
- Castor sugar
- Coconut palm sugar
- Coconut sugar
- Confectioner's sugar
- Corn sweetener
- Corn syrup
- Corn syrup solids
- Date sugar
- Dehydrated cane juice
- Demerara sugar
- Dextrin
- Dextrose
- Evaporated cane juice
- Free-flowing brown sugars
- Fructose
- Fruit juice
- Fruit juice concentrate
- Glucose
- Glucose solids
- Golden sugar
- Golden syrup
- Grape sugar
- HFCS (High-Fructose Corn Syrup)
- Honey
- Icing sugar
- Invert sugar

- Malt syrup
- Maltodextrin
- Maltol
- Maltose
- Mannose
- Maple syrup
- Molasses
- Muscovado
- Palm sugar
- Panocha
- Powdered sugar
- Raw sugar
- Refiner's syrup
- Rice syrup
- Saccharose
- Sorghum Syrup
- Sucrose
- Sugar (granulated)
- Sweet Sorghum
- Syrup
- Treacle
- Turbinado sugar
- Yellow sugar

https://www.healthline.com/nutrition/too-much-sugar
https://www.healthline.com/nutrition/how-much-sugar-per-day

28

There is More to It Than Just the Number on the Scale

HEN YOU CHANGE WHAT YOU EAT WITH AN EMPHASIS on consuming more vegetables and protein (baked chicken and turkey, baked fish, beans) and less starches and sugar, your body composition predictably will change over time. You may notice a change in your muscle tone and the location on your body where you have fat deposited within 2-3 months of sticking to your plan. This is especially true if you are exercising as well.

Because muscle is heavier and denser than fat, your weight on the scale may not decrease quickly, may plateau at some point, and may even increase. This should NOT be a cause for despair. Muscle is metabolically healthier and more efficient with respect to how you metabolize what you eat. Metabolism "is the internal process by which your body expends energy and burns calories. It runs 24/7 to keep your body moving, even when you're resting or sleeping, by converting the food and nutrients you consume into the energy your body needs in order to breathe, circulate blood, grow and repair cells, and everything else it does to survive." (https://www.health.harvard.edu/staying-healthy/the-truth-about-metabolism)

I encourage patients not to weigh themselves until they come in the office, if weighing at home will discourage them. Your body fat and muscle composition are altered when you change eating habits and subsequently begin to lose weight. The number that you see on the scale may not adequately reflect everything that is going on inside your body with respect to the change in your metabolism.

A more useful and informative way to evaluate your weight loss efforts and metabolic progress is to measure your loss in inches and to do body fat analysis. You can simply measure arm, thigh and waist circumference if you don't have a digital scale that does body fat analysis or skin fold calipers or have access to a gym or university fitness center that has body fat analysis equipment. Your loss of inches in these areas of the body indicates that you are becoming leaner, and you are replacing fat with muscle.

BODY FAT ANALYSIS

- In general, body fat should be:
  - Women <32%
  - Men <25%
- Body fat analysis scale-readily available in many current home weight scales
- Body circumference-measuring inches around the mid-upper arm, around the belly button and the mid-thigh
- Measuring skinfold thickness of mid-upper arm, mid-abdomen and mid-thigh with calipers-can be done by yourself or by a fitness trainer

- Underwater measurement (hydrodensitometry)-available at many retail and university fitness centers that have a pool
- Air displacement/Bod Pod (air displacement plethysmograph)-available in many retail fitness centers and university fitness centers around the country
- https://www.healthline.com/health/exercise-fitness/ideal-body-fat-percentage
- https://www.healthline.com/nutrition/ways-to-measure-body-fat
- https://www.xyngular.com/en/blog/how-to-measure-weight-loss-without-a-scale/
- https://www.cosmed.com/en/contact-us/test-site-locator

Whatever method you use, the decrease in your numbers (weight, inches, body fat percentage) over time is more important than the accuracy of the method that you use.

Body Mass Index or BMI takes into account what your weight should be based on your height. https://www.cdc.gov/healthyweight/assessing/bmi/adult_bmi/english_bmi_calculator/bmi_calculator.html

BMI (body mass index) recommendations about what is actually appropriate weight:

MALE					
AGE	EXCELLENT 1	VERY GOOD 2	GOOD 3	FAIR 4	POOR 5
19–24	< 11	11.1–15	15.1–19	19.1–23	> 23
25–29	< 13	13.1–17	17.1–20	20.1–24	> 24
30–34	< 15	15.1–18	18.1–22	22.1–25	> 25

MALE					
AGE	EXCELLENT 1	VERY GOOD 2	GOOD 3	FAIR 4	POOR 5
35–39	< 16	16.1–19	19.1–23	23.1–26	> 26
40–44	< 18	18.1–21	21.1–24	24.1–27	> 27
45–49	< 19	19.1–22	22.1–25	25.1–28	> 28
50–54	< 20	22.1–23	23.1–26	26.1–29	> 29
55+	< 21	20.1–24	24.1–27	27.1–30	> 30

FEMALE					
AGE	EXCELLENT 1	VERY GOOD 2	GOOD 3	FAIR 4	POOR 5
19–24	< 19	19.1–22	22.1–25	25.1–30	> 30
25–29	< 19	19.1–22	22.1–25	25.1–30	> 30
30–34	< 20	20.1–23	23.1–26	26.1–31	> 31
35–39	< 21	21.1–24	24.1–28	28.1–32	> 32
40–44	< 23	23.1–26	26.1–29	29.1–33	> 33
45–49	< 24	24.1–27	27.1–31	31.1–34	> 34
50–54	< 27	27.1–31	31.1–34	34.1–37	> 37
55+	< 28	28.1–31	31.1–34	34.1–38	> 38

Current guidelines say that you should strive to have a BMI of less than 25, in general, however we are moving toward a recalibration of BMI values that defines obesity in a more biologically based approach, (which) allows for a more individualized approach rather than the current "one-size fits all." https://www.mayoclinicproceedings.org/article/S0025-6196(18)30807-3/fulltext

TABLE. Cutoffs for BMI Based on ROC Curve Analysis						
	BMI (kg/m^2)					
	Men			Women		
Obesity Co-morbidity	Black	Hispanic	White	Black	Hispanic	White
Hypertension	28	29	28	31	28	27
Dyslipidemia	27	26	27	29	27	25
Diabetes	29	29	30	33	30	29
≥2 risk factors	28	29	29	31	30	28
Average	28	28	29	31	29	27

BMI = body mass index; ROC = receiver operating characteristic.

29

Look Outside How You Feel Inside

A PATIENT SAID TO ME ONE DAY, "I WANT TO LOOK OUTSIDE how I feel inside," when expressing her desire to lose weight. She was a relatively new patient to my practice and seemed to be a level-headed and satisfied person. She was frustrated with her inability to lose weight and needed some guidance to move toward her health and weight loss goals. Her statement was a reminder for me that not everybody who is overweight is unhappy or depressed or has underlying issues that are blocking the path to their success in losing weight to get to their desired goal. For a lot of people, being overweight has its roots in psychological barriers that need to be addressed, but for others, it is not a matter of being sad or depressed. Many people who are overweight are NOT emotional eaters. For many, the situation is not very complicated and only a matter of just needing guidance, instruction, and accountability about what to eat and how often to eat. Many people do not know what healthy food choices are and simple education about making better decisions through reading labels can get them to their goals in a short period of time.

YOUR MENTAL HEALTH CONTROLS
YOUR PHYSICAL HEALTH

*There are many colorful flowers on the path of life, but
the prettiest have the sharpest thorns.*
African Proverb

Life is lived forwards, but understood backwards.
African Proverb

*Worry is like a rocking chair; it swings you back and
forth and it takes you nowhere.*
African Proverb

30

Regretitis™

WOULDA, SHOULDA, COULDA.

Regretitis™ is a term I made up to describe a chronic and sometimes deadly condition that occurs when a person ruminates over choices he or she has made during their lives they now regret. This may seem like a funny term, but I coined it for myself to describe a serious chronic condition I have come to notice and address with patients. Not missing this "diagnosis" can be the difference between enjoying life and a slow death for a patient. This primarily applies to decisions that people make when they had other options and later regret the choice. Unfortunately, there are many decisions that people make that have negative long-term consequences and cannot be reversed. Sometimes these choices are decisions made as young adults that, in retrospect, were ill-advised.

Over the course of taking care of a person as their primary care physician, I get to learn about the choices that people regret because they communicate these feelings to me when past choices are affecting their current physical and mental health.

Life choices that people make that intersect with current and future health include:

- Choice of spouse or significant other
- Relationship choices
- Education, business, and career choices
- Decision to have or not have children
- Decisions made that affect pregnancy and birth outcomes
- Child-rearing decisions
- Chronic disease management decisions -- lack of decision or ignoring chronic diseases over many years leading to disease complications
- Not seeking treatment for mental health conditions leading to mental health challenges
- Not communicating with someone prior to their death
- Not communicating feelings with someone who is still living
- Not following good advice when it was given
- Choice of people allowed into inner circle in life

Many patients become chronically despondent because no amount of contemplation or reflection about the past choice(s) changes the present. It is a very insidious state of mind such that people can spiral downward and into a persistent state of hopelessness and despair. Patients can get to a point where they cannot let go of, reconcile, or accept the past in order to be able to move forward. This state of mind can often affect those closest to the patient. Regretitis ™ in a patient can translate to despair because no one can help the patient out of their condition.

Patients are often so shrouded and cloaked in remorse that their current decisions are clouded by their underlying mental state. It is challenging to help patients maintain their health and control chronic medical conditions when regretitis ™ has firmly established itself within the patient. This condition causes people to have difficulty attending to the present because the past haunts them significantly.

We all have made choices in life, large and small, that we wish we could take back. But the hands of time cannot be reversed and being paralyzed by consequences of the past can compound current problems in whole and in part, by past decisions. We have to forgive ourselves for past actions and/or inactions in order to free ourselves from the personal health inertia that regretitis ™ causes. I have seen patients' lives transformed when they finally let go of things, people, and circumstances they cannot change and start to live for today and tomorrow. Doing this releases a larger burden for the patient, and they become more engaged in their own health care and become better advocates for themselves.

I had a longstanding patient who was essentially consumed by his thoughts about his mother who repeatedly, from his 20's until current day, expressed to him her disappointment that he did not have a career as a professional athlete. Much of his daily life thoughts and actions were paralyzed by his distress with his mother's lack of support for his life trajectory that led him to a career in science. I encouraged him to consider accepting his mother as she is but not let her words continue to haunt him because it was causing anxiety and impairing his ability to maintain his health because he could not make healthy choices about what he ate, follow instructions about taking his medications, and do his home self-monitoring for his high blood pressure and diabetes. His poor disease management was making him at risk for heart and kidney disease in the near future. I also encouraged him to start counseling to help him manage his anxiety.

After several visits discussing this, he told me he started counseling and was beginning to feel better about himself in dealing with his feelings about his mother. He began to do much better with checking his blood pressure and glucose at home, making healthier food choices, and his diabetes and blood pressure control has improved significantly.

Check with your insurance company to see what your mental health benefits are. Many have behavioral health networks and case managers to facilitate getting mental health counseling and psychiatric services, which are now not as limited by location due to insurance companies now paying for video visits.

31

You Don't Have to Feel This Way

O NE TYPICAL DAY, A PATIENT SAID TO ME, "I DECIDED THAT I don't have to feel this way," at a visit that she scheduled to discuss how she was feeling. She initially declined treatment for depression and anxiety at her previous visit, but one week later sent me a patient portal message saying she wanted medication to treat her anxiety and depression. She made this statement when I asked her what made her change her mind. She said that she was "just tired of feeling bad" and wanted to do something about it. Her non-medication ways of managing her depression and anxiety were not working. She concluded that her ways of managing anxiety and stress had never worked and she wanted to try medication. She expressed she was denying herself the ability to try available treatment options that other people were availing themselves of and getting better. The patient had already done many therapy trials as an adult but was always reluctant to try medication when it was recommended.

Social, environmental, and genetic issues can influence a person's mental health status and the need for behavioral health evaluation. Maximizing mental health beyond these uncontrollable factors by engaging in healthy eating, getting enough sleep, and getting regular exercise are at the foundation of improving mental health status. I typically stress to my patients that medication for depression and anxiety is only one prong of a multi-pronged approach to managing anxiety and depression.

Taking medication as an adjunct to non-medication modalities to treat anxiety and depression can help patients feel better and improve the quality of their lives. Medication for depression and anxiety does not have to be taken indefinitely but can be at least taken long enough to improve how one feels. Medication can be taken for 3-12 months and then discontinued with supervision by the doctor, monitoring for recurrence of symptoms.

In addition, I always recommend establishing care with a therapist, psychologist and/or psychiatrist to help with therapy in conjunction with prescribing medication. Often patients may have more complicated psychiatric issues and conditions that need care by a trained mental health/behavioral health professional. Often patients have multiple psychiatric conditions going on at the same time and this can be evaluated and diagnosed by a trained professional.

Medication side effects can occur, but they can be managed or medication type and/or dose adjustments can be done to maximize effectiveness and limit side effects. In general, medications currently used for the treatment for anxiety and depression do not affect the function of internal organs significantly. Regular follow up with your doctor for medication surveillance will lead to minimal problems with taking these types of medications.

These are some common medications used to treat anxiety and depression. This is not an exhaustive list, but these are medications that people hear about or know about someone else taking:

- Zoloft (Sertraline)
- Effexor (Venlafaxine)
- Paxil (Paroxetine)
- Prozac (Fluoxetine)
- Lexapro (Escitalopram)

- Wellbutrin (Bupropion)
- Celexa (Citalopram)
- Cymbalta (Duloxetine)

Taking medication for psychiatric conditions is not an admission of a flaw in character or personal failing. Feeling bad, feeling down, feeling sad, depressed, and being anxious are common ways of feeling, but these symptoms do not have to be disruptive, dysfunctional and are an inevitable part of life. These symptoms can be evaluated and treated just like physical and medical conditions are treated.

32

Don't Get Stuck in Your Thoughts

A PATIENT SAID THIS TO ME DURING A VISIT ONE DAY when she was telling me about how she works with herself to manage her anxiety and depression without medication. She told me that she manages her symptoms of anxiety and depression by being aware of her thoughts and making sure that she did not let herself ruminate on negative thoughts. She said that doing this requires that a person to be very aware of their thinking on a second-by-second, minute-by-minute and hour-by-hour basis. She said that over time, it gets easier to become self-aware of day-to-day feelings and well-being, which helps alleviate the symptoms of anxiety and depression.

Symptoms that could be anxiety and depression include:

- Excessive worrying
- Physical symptoms like sweating and muscle tension, headache, pain in the neck, shoulders, and back
- Difficulty falling asleep and difficulty staying asleep

- Sleeping too much
- Fatigue
- Difficulty relaxing
- Depressed mood, like feeling down, feeling sad, feeling empty, hopelessness, tearful a lot
- Decrease interest or pleasure in daily activities
- Weight loss that is not intended
- Decreased appetite
- Feeling of loss of energy
- Feeling hyperactive
- Feelings of worthlessness
- Excessive feelings of guilt
- Decrease ability to concentrate and/or make decisions
- Fear of dying
- Frequent thoughts about death
- Thoughts about ending one's life (committing suicide)

Ultimately, many of these symptoms can be managed without medication. Primary care physician or mental health provider consultation should be done first to have these symptoms evaluated to see if emergent and urgent treatment is needed. THINKING OF ENDING ONE'S LIFE IS AN EMERGENCY.

At a conference, I learned about this simple way to check in with yourself on a regular, even daily basis, to stay in touch with how you are feeling and having a plan to help yourself when emotions start to be overwhelming.

MY WELLNESS PLAN

These are signs that I am feeling down, sad or not myself:

_____

These are things that I can try to help me feel better:

_____

I normally find joy in these things because:

_____

When I am feeling down, sad, or not myself, the person my age I can talk to is:

_____

When I am feeling down, sad, or not myself, the website, app, phone number I will call/text is:

_____

When I am feeling down, sad, or not myself, another adult that I can talk to is:

_____

33

The Two Letter Word

$\mathcal{I}$ HAVE COME TO ADVISE PATIENTS TO DEVELOP A STRONG command of the use of the word "NO". Often patients are in situations in their lives where they have trouble saying NO to friends and family when they are asked for favors, asked to perform duties and tasks for others. People may have just a gratuitous nature or may feel obligated to grant requests on their time and finances. Patients can become overwhelmed, overworked, overstressed with trying to fulfill the duties they've taken upon themselves. This is especially true with younger patients who have yet to become comfortable with using the word NO when things are asked of them. In addition, the word NO is difficult for many to use because of fear of the requester being angry with them if the request is not granted.

I remember a patient who had taken on being the primary caregiver for a friend who had multiple chronic medical conditions and who needed lots of supervision with taking her medications, care at home, and transportation to her multiple medical visits. This was increasingly becoming a burden, and she expressed her desire to relinquish the responsibility of her friend's care to her family. Her friend had lots of willing family to help with her care but chose to call upon my patient to help her instead. My patient told me that, although she felt no particular obligation to her friend, she just couldn't say no when her friend called for help and assistance. My patient had begun to neglect her own personal obligations with her own family and her own health as her friend's medical care became more complicated.

We discussed the implications of her starting to use the word NO with her friend and my patient told me reluctantly that she would consider trying to say no. We discussed this over a few visits and one visit she told me that she had begun to follow my advice, and she was doing less for her friend. She was able to attend to her own health and she was getting caught up on the orders, referrals and preventive health tests that I had been reminding her about, which led to her health improving. Her friend's family had taken over the responsibility of her care and my patient was still able to contribute to her friend, but in a lesser degree than before. My patient felt better, less stressed, and was still able to maintain her friendship.

Sometimes saying NO can cost a friendship or can have a negative effect on relationships as a consequence, but sometimes this is something that is inevitable when others are repeatedly demanding of your efforts and time. It can be very liberating to be able to comfortably use the word NO as one matures in life and to still be OK when people become indignant and maybe even angry when their requests are not granted.

The most common situation where I am having this conversation is with patients who are taking care of grandchildren, men and women alike, because the adult parent(s) have abdicated their obligations of parenthood and the responsibility has been taken on by the grandparents. Where one or more parents have passed away or they have a mental disability or physical/medical issue that prevents them from taking care of the children, it is understandable grandparents would step into this role. But this is often not the case.

This situation is often very stressful for people who are aging, less active, less able to maintain the rigors of child-rearing, including providing housing, clothing, food, and taking minors to medical appointments. It is especially challenging when the patients themselves have their own set of progressive medical conditions and physician appointments.

The conversation with a patient about this predicament often comes up when a patient is not taking care of themselves with respect to eating healthy, exercising, taking prescribed medications, and going to specialist appointments. The patient invariably expresses extreme frustration with being unable to do the tasks needed for their own health. I often ask, "Where are the parents of these children?" The answer is usually that the parents are not responsible, and the patient has taken on child-rearing because the patient wants to make sure that the children get appropriate care.

Often grandparent primary care giving occurs after the threat of foster care has ensued. The patient often despairs with the fact they feel their adult child is taking advantage of them instead of raising their own children. Often it is the grandmother that is reluctant to relinquish care of the child back to their parent(s) because of fear the child will again not be well cared for, like when the child (ren) came to them initially. I have had many patients that are grandmothers who have raised grandchildren from birth and the parents of these children have never been involved in their care. Patients may acknowledge their adult child has had a lifetime of being irresponsible and the lack of taking on the responsibility of parenting is just another manifestation of their negligence. There are often feelings of guilt associated with this phenomenon.

I have often had to encourage my patients to relinquish care or decrease caregiving duties and responsibilities so they can attend to their own health. For many, this is a difficult decision to make and often my patient has to relinquish care because their own health is so bad they can no longer continue raising their grandchildren.

34

Change Your Expectation of a Perfect Life

*T*HE DISCUSSION ABOUT LIFE EXPECTATIONS FREQUENTLY comes up during my visits with patients when their health is not optimal. I find that many patients are tormented as they go through life because they are disappointed their life didn't turn out the way they wanted it to. I think that as a society, we have an unrealistic expectation of what life is supposed to be. I see this issue as being more uniquely American, as many patients I've had over the years who were not born in this country have a different way of looking at life.

Life issues that patients often acknowledge they've have had idealistic expectations about:

- Who would they marry?
- Success of romantic relationships
- Success of family relationships
- How much money they can make
- Having children

- Not having children
- What their children would achieve in life
- Expectations about health
- Expectations about mental health

I feel that many of us expect life to happen the way we want, when we want it, without us guiding what we want to happen in our lives and/or making choices that will lead to the outcome that we want in life. Patients who have difficulty with reconciling their lives with what they expected from life can create this insidious condition of regretitis™ that I detailed above.

35

The Hardships in Life That Prevent People from Focusing on Their Health

*T*HERE IS AN EXTENSIVE LIST OF LIFE HARDSHIPS AND personal stressors that patients tell me about that prevents them from focusing on their health. Here are some of the common ones:

- Work stress
- Raising children
- Relationship and marital stress
- Family stress
- Taking care of elderly parents
- Taking care of grandchildren
- Lack of insurance and being under-insured
- Financial stress
- Financial obligations

- Not having enough income to support everyday needs of the patient and/or family
- Having to work long hours
- Having multiple jobs to make ends meet
- Not getting enough sleep due to life responsibilities
- Being overextended with responsibilities in life that are either chosen or not chosen

I allow patients to express their frustrations about the discordance of their actual vs. ideal life standing. Patients appreciate the opportunity to talk about their life challenges, as most don't have a chance to vent elsewhere in their lives. I typically don't hear their entire life story during any one visit, but I get to hear about their life challenges over the course of our relationship. I used to feel compelled to solve all their problems and often felt helpless when I could not. But I have come to learn that patients do not expect me to solve their problems, but they use the time in the doctor's office to be able to vent and express their frustrations. I now focus on how I can tailor my recommendations for their health to accommodate their life challenges or encourage them to empower themselves to change what they can change and want to change in their lives such that they can progress toward their health care goals.

36

How Social Media Can Hinder Health and Well Being

*T*HESE DAYS, MANY PEOPLE ARE STRESSED OUT BY THE STATE of the world and the situation in this country that they see on television and on social media every day. The pandemic that started in 2020 has heightened the level of stress of all of us. Stress that comes from social media is a real entity, and I have had a multitude of discussions with patients regarding stressful situations, negative thoughts about life status and self-worth that have arisen from social media drama and reading what other people post on social media. People can be unduly distressed about their own lives when seeing what is posted by others on social media. I frequently have to remind people that what people post about their lives on social media is often overinflated and that one cannot judge their own life based on what someone else "says" their life is.

In addition, there is a lot of misinformation on social media about what is and *is not* healthy and often patients come to me asking about supplements and fad diets and treatments that I do not recommend. I advise people that I do not feel strongly about supplements above eating lots of fruits and vegetables in their diet. Supplements are meant to supplement holes in your nutrition. If you do not have holes in your nutrition, then you do not need supplements. Intermittent fasting is a method of eating that patients are reading a lot about on social media. I encourage patients to eat during the day, while awake, as you have suffi-cient "fasting" with the recommended amount of sleep. (Shahada Karim, Habbi Body Sport https://www.habibibodysport.com/)

37

Worrying About Things That You Have No Control Over Can Make You Sick or Kill You

DON'T WORRY ABOUT THINGS THAT YOU CAN DO NOTHING about.

Asking patients, "What are you most worried about?" can bring to light unspoken concerns and allow fears to be addressed.

I see a lot of patients who worry about things they have no control over instead of focusing on the things they do have control over. The main thing we all have control over for the most part is what we eat and how much exercise we get. These two things are not trivial aspects in our lives that can be very impactful when done consistently. Even for people who live in areas that we now call food deserts (I call them healthy food deserts -- there is often plenty of food available, but much of it is not healthy) can still be cognizant of making as healthy food choices as possible. Even in the suburbs, there are a plethora of restaurants and fast-food places, such that quick, unhealthy food choices are much easier to choose than healthier ones.

I support the notion that it is not constructive to worry about diseases and medical conditions that could develop where we have no way to diagnose early. Many human illnesses have causes we have no control over, may not have a good treatment for and cannot find before it becomes a problem. This is a fact that I have come to accept as a physician, but a concept that is difficult for many of us to accept. Another issue that I discuss with patients is the futility of worrying about other people's behaviors which we have no control over. This is a common issue when a patient is dealing with the behavior of adult children, parents, co-workers, friends, spouses, and significant others that is affecting their health.

Patients often have physical symptoms due to anxiety that stem, in whole or in part, from the unknown factors in our environment (medical illness, pandemic infections, climate instability and political strife, etc.) and the complicated world that we live in. I see a lot of patients who have physical symptoms from stress and anxiety that often need treatment, including counseling and/or medication. Chronic worry can turn into a significant variable with respect to improving a medical condition or constellation of symptoms.

I strive to educate patients to understand that good health, maintenance of health, disease prevention, and prevention of disease progression is an active process and not just a matter of being a passive participant in their own health. I try to push patients to be active participants in their health, including encouraging home self-monitoring if they have high blood pressure or diabetes, encouraging patients to do food diaries for us to review to help the patient make themselves accountable to themselves instead of just being accountable to me as their primary care physician. I find that once I can change the patient's mindset about being an active participant in their own healthcare and holding themselves accountable, they actually feel more empowered and more in control of things they can control instead of feeling helpless from the many things that we do not have control over in our lives.

38

Lost Sleep is Just That.... Lost!

G ETTING ENOUGH RESTORATIVE SLEEP IS CRUCIAL FOR good health. Once you miss out on sleep, you can't fully make up for it later by just sleeping more. For many, work and personal duties inhibit people from getting into the bed. Commonly, I discuss a patient's inability to allow their thoughts to rest once they lie down to rest. People can have trouble falling asleep, staying asleep and can have sleep related disorders that impair the sleep cycle. I recommend that any problem with sleeping be investigated by the primary care physician and referral to a sleep specialist and/or mental health provider may be warranted for further evaluation. Keeping a diary of sleep patterns and habits can be very useful in trying to reveal a dysfunctional sleep pattern or cause of sleep trouble.

Here is a list of questions that I have patients answer to try to assess the nature of their problem with sleeping:

- Are you having trouble falling asleep, staying asleep, or both?
- How long does it take for you to fall asleep?

- Do you snore loudly?
- Has anyone ever told you that you stop breathing while you are asleep?
- Are you tired during the day?
- Do you nap during the day?
- Do you drink coffee or alcohol?
- If you wake up after going to sleep, do you go back to sleep easily?
- What wakes you up from sleep?
- What do you do on the nights you cannot sleep?
- What time do you get in bed?
- What time do you get out of bed?
- Do you have worries and/or anxiety about sleep?

Sleep hygiene/healthy sleep habits/things to try to help with sleep:

- No television in the bedroom.
- Avoid daytime sleeping and afternoon naps.
- Regular exercise 4-5 hours before bedtime will help with sleep, but do not exercise close to bedtime.
- No heavy meals within 3 hours of bedtime.
- Do not drink alcohol within a few hours of bedtime and limit the use of alcohol altogether.
- Avoid caffeine in the evening and consider avoiding ALL caffeine.
- If you are unable to fall asleep within 20 minutes, get out of bed and do something else until sleepy (cleaning, reading a book, etc.). Repeat the cycle until sleep occurs.
- Limit light exposure 3 hours prior to bedtime, especially television, computer and tablet watching.

- Avoid excessive light exposure when trying to go to sleep, i.e. turn off or dim all lights, clocks, personal devices that emit light; use room darkening curtains/shades.
- Provide yourself generous light exposure upon awakening. Sunlight is best.
- Establish a sleep routine. Regular bed and wake times amounting to 7-8 hours per 24-hour period.
- Complete smoking cessation is recommended for overall health, including sleep health.
- Exercise daily. 20-30 minutes a day can help you sleep more soundly.
- Avoid strenuous exercise 1 hour before bedtime.
- Try relaxation activities prior to bedtime.

Cognitive therapy thoughts and techniques that can help with sleep:

- Daytime sleepiness symptoms are not always a consequence of poor sleep.
- Reduce unrealistic expectations regarding sleep. Your poor sleep is not as bad as you think.
- Improve your perception of sleep to avoid over generalizations, ruminations and exaggerations associated with sleep.
- Work on mindfulness and positive thinking at bedtime to reduce your sleep anxiety.
- Stimulus control therapy
- Lie down intending to go to sleep only when you are sleepy.
- Do not use your bed for anything except sleep. The thinking behind this is to promote behavior modification such

that you are trying to train your brain to associate the bed only with sleep. This is key for people who have problems sleeping.

- If you are unable to fall asleep within 10 minutes, get up and go through another dark room and sit quietly.
- Return to lying down to sleep and repeat as many times as necessary.

https://www.sleepfoundation.org/insomnia/treatment/cognitive-behavioral-therapy-insomnia
https://stanfordhealthcare.org/medical-treatments/c/cognitive-behavioral-therapy-insomnia/procedures/stimulus-control.html

Relaxation techniques to be done 30 minutes prior to bedtime that can help promote sleep:

- Progressive muscle relaxation: 5-second tensing and relaxing of muscle groups from head to toe. You can find the instructions on how to do this on many websites.
- Guided imagery: Looking at calm nature scenes while listening to music.
- Abdominal breathing: Breathing and slowly through your nose, allowing your chest and lower belly to rise as you feel your lungs. Your abdomen expands fully. Then, breathe out slowly through your mouth. Repeat several times.
- Repeat a favorite mantra to yourself at bedtime.
- Meditation and mindfulness is helpful at bedtime.
- Mindfulness practices can help with muscle tension, anxiety, sleep, chronic pain, headaches and many other

medical conditions. Yoga is one example of mindfulness practice. Yoga can be done in classes but there are DVD and online options for learning how to do yoga.

- Guided meditations in short sessions of 10-20 minutes are another form of mindfulness that can be helpful. Some helpful smartphone apps include "Stop, Think and Breathe," "Insight Timer," and "Calm."

I do not recommend medication for sleep very often, as they can disrupt sleep even more in the long run. I can recommend these to help promote sleep (check with your doctor to make sure that these are safe for you): Sleepy Time tea, chamomile tea, Valerian root tea, and melatonin supplement at bedtime.

39

Don't Create a Loneliness Bubble

$\mathcal{I}$ HAD A PATIENT SAY THIS TO ME ONE DAY WHEN TALKING about how she must sometimes rely on others to help her with health issues, as medical conditions started to manifest themselves or become diagnosed. Her observation was that often she sees that people alienate others in their earlier lives and end up with having no one to help them with their activities of daily living, health care and medical needs, when they occur. I have seen this play out in many patients' lives during my career.

A lot of times patients develop medical problems where they slowly lose their independence, their ability to take care of themselves and keep up with their medical issues. They may find themselves without assistance because they have alienated friends and family for a multitude of reasons. I am using the word "alienated", but my patient used the terms "piss people off", "made people mad", which I further interpreted to mean "being disagreeable with others", "mistreating others" such that the person has "burned all of their bridges" to anyone who would have been available and willing to help them with medical concerns, transportation to doctors' appointments, outpatient diagnostic procedures and/or testing, helping clean the house, and helping them manage and keep up with taking their medications properly to name a few. A typical story is that the patient has a pervasive history such that they have slowly alienated people in their lives and usually not because of any type of mental illness or mental health disorder. In fact, often, patients with mental health disorders do in fact have someone who is willing to step up and take care of them (or a legal guardian has been in place long ago) as opposed to those who just have a challenging personality and are basically difficult to get along with according to their friends and family.

Often there are insurance constraints and lack of community resources to take the place of the gaps in care that friends and families can fill. Patients who are in this situation are a challenge to take care of because family and friends are often much better resources for assistance than trying to find community and agency resources to fulfill this role. This all means that I will find that friends and family are not willing to help with the care of the patient when asked by the patient, myself, or someone from the medical office. Situations like this can become very dire to the point that a legal guardian must be obtained for the patient so someone can oversee their care and make life choices for them because they can no longer do it for themselves.

In addition, friends and family who have been mistreated in the past often can often be vengeful, spiteful, and retaliatory to the patient who has mistreated them. The abuse is in the form of neglect more than anything else. I have had situations where Adult Protective Services needed to be contacted to protect the patient from abusive or neglectful friends and family members.

I remember a new elderly patient whose brother was not bringing him to his scheduled appointments. When the patient was brought to his appointments, he was always unkempt, did not smell good, had on dirty clothes, and looked like he was not eating enough. He always had a despondent look on his face. The patient was functional (able to walk, talk and feed himself, but needed help with grooming and personal hygiene), but he told me that he was financially dependent on his brother for his housing, food, and transportation. I discussed this at an early visit with the patient and he told me that he could only provide for himself what his brother provided for him. He also told me that his brother was obstructing his ability to leave his home and live with his sister. I was able to speak to the patient's brother once, and he communicated that he did not have a good relationship with the patient and felt resentful about caring for his brother because of past mistreatment from the patient, going back to their early adulthood.

I contacted the local APS, and they were able to facilitate getting the patient out of the home with his son and into a safe and nurturing environment with the patient's sister. He was able to access his medical benefits and have control of his personal finances. The patient never looked disheveled again after he moved out of his brother's home. After that, he came to all of his scheduled appointments, looked happier and developed a healthier weight and overall well-being.

How you treat others earlier in life can be returned to you later in life when you need someone. This concept includes helping others when you're able to, because those people are very likely to help you later in life when you need them.

Some may call this Karma!

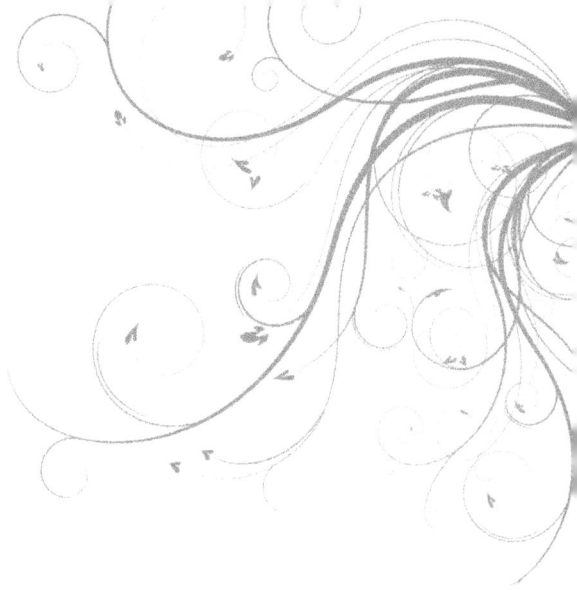

For the Ladies

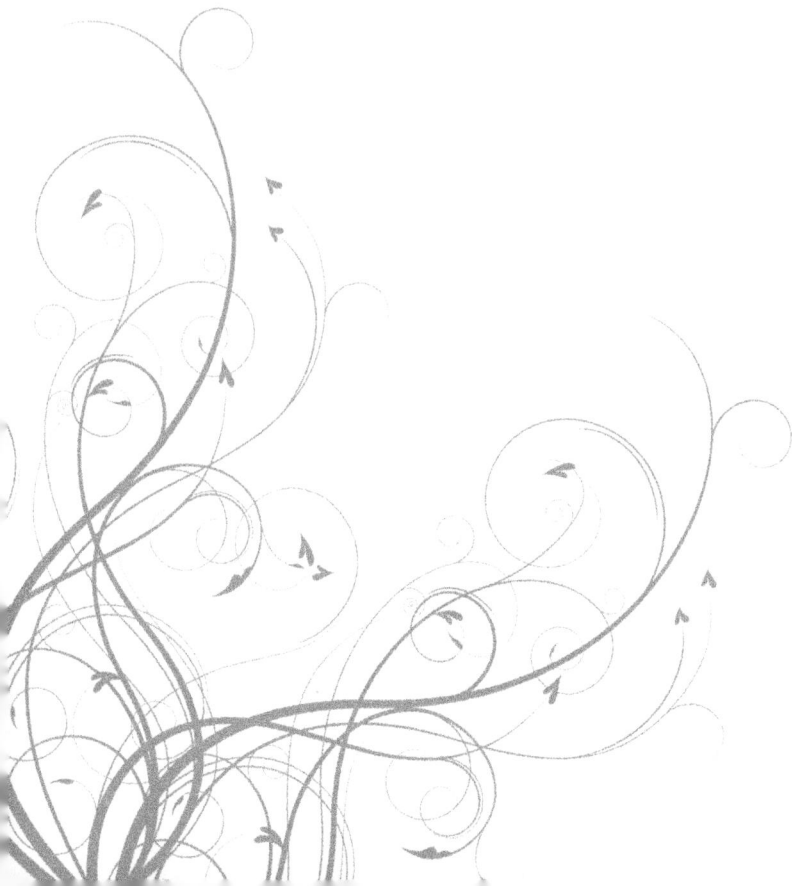

40

Connection Between Stress and Anxiety and Vaginal Bacterial Overgrowth and Vaginal Candida (Yeast) Overgrowth

ANY CONCERN ABOUT VAGINAL SYMPTOMS SHOULD BE evaluated by your primary care physician or your gynecologist (GYN).

I have come to observe a correlation between the overgrowth of vaginal yeast and vaginal bacteria conditions in women and increased stress in a woman's life and/or environment.

Many women know these symptoms as a "yeast infection" or a "bacterial infection" (bacterial vaginosis or BV).

The vaginal symptoms of:

- A change from the usual vaginal smell or odor
- Any vaginal itching

- An increase in the usual vaginal discharge and/or vaginal output

These conditions are not really "infections," but rather they occur when a change in the environment or acidity level of the vagina creates an atmosphere in the vagina where there is an overgrowth of vaginal yeast and/or vaginal bacteria that normally lives in the vagina at controlled levels. Therefore, I call the conditions "overgrowth" instead of "infections." An infection is the invasion and multiplication of microorganisms such as bacteria, viruses, and parasites that are not normally present within the body. An infection may cause no symptoms and be subclinical, or it may cause symptoms and be clinically apparent.

I have come to routinely ask female patients about stress in their lives when they report a change in their vaginal function or report new and/or recurrent vaginal symptoms. The vagina should have a usual output/discharge and odor. Vaginal itching is never normal and should always be evaluated for other causes other than yeast and bacterial overgrowth. The overgrowth of vaginal yeast and bacteria that normally is there can cause discomfort, itching, change in vaginal odor and increased vaginal discharge. I educate female patients about the correlation between vaginal symptoms and stress to make them aware that emotional stress coming from their everyday life and/or environment should be addressed, so they can modify their behavior and/or modify their environment to decrease stress and control symptoms.

I have had many patients who have come to have much less frequent or no further vaginal yeast and bacteria overgrowth symptoms after they have made life changes to relieve stress (changes in family dynamics, counseling, changing jobs or em-ployment/career situations).

Although effective treatments are available to control vaginal yeast and vaginal bacterial overgrowth, controlling and having a plan of response to stress in life can contribute to having a more favorable vaginal environment.

41

Women Take Care of Everyone but Themselves

$\mathcal{I}$ HAVE ALSO OBSERVED THAT WOMEN HAVE A BAD HABIT OF taking care of the needs of others above their own:

- Spouse/significant other
- Children
- Siblings
- Grandchildren

Many women are unaware they are more focused on taking care of others and forsaking their own care. I often have to bring this to their attention when I observe behaviors that are detrimental to their own health:

- Missing primary care and specialist appointments
- Forgetting to refill prescription medications
- Eating on the go and not planning to eat healthy foods
- Not cooking or eating foods cooked from home
- Not getting labs draws and diagnostic testing done when ordered

- Not getting preventive health tests done when ordered (mammogram, colonoscopy, etc.)
- Ignoring symptoms and/or prolonging seeking medical care for evaluation of symptoms
- Not returning phone calls or responding to patient portal messages from the doctor's office
- Not following instructions about taking medications or changes in medications
- Not seeing a specialist when referred to do so

When I brought this issue to the attention of a patient during a visit one day (she had not done her mammogram and had missed several appointments), she said that she had not done what she was supposed to do for herself because, "I am so busy running around for everyone else!" She then got quiet and proceeded to tell me that she had not even realized how much she was neglecting herself. The conversation with this patient has been echoed repeatedly by so many other female patients over the course of my career.

42

"A Call from the Bladder is Louder Than a King's Command"

THIS IS A PHRASE THAT I HAVE HEARD FROM MY MOTHER for as long as I remember. She would make this statement often when she had delayed going to the bathroom to empty her bladder and was at risk of having an "accident" if she didn't get to the bathroom soon. Of note, my mother is a retired teacher. I came to observe that my female patients who are currently teachers frequently told me about how they delay bladder emptying because their opportunities to go to the bathroom are decreased because their classroom duties prevent them from leaving the classroom full of children to go empty their bladder when it "calls." These conversations typically occur when I am evaluating their complaints related to having:

- Urinary frequency
- Waking up at night too much to urinate

- Leaking of urine
- Leaking of urine with coughing, laughing, and sneezing
- Losing control of the ability to hold urine in the bladder, urine "accidents"

Bladder symptoms should always be evaluated, as there are many possible causes. However, I advise all patients to heed the call from the bladder, because bladder muscle tone can be decreased over many years when a person allows the bladder to stay full without emptying, ignoring the sensation that occurs when the bladder is "calling".

Over time, I have coined to myself the term, "teacher's bladder", referring to a female patient who has the onset of bladder symptoms, who were also classroom teachers and tell me that they have a long-time habit of holding their urine because they cannot leave their classroom as they would like. I smile to myself when addressing the patient's complaints because it makes me think of my mother.

Epilogue

If I Were in Charge of Everything Tomorrow

D EALING WITH THE WORLD WE LIVE IN CAN OFTEN BE very frustrating for me as a person and as a doctor trying to help my patients. I brought up this topic with a patient one day while we were sharing our frustrations about the challenges we all encounter in today's society, especially concerning affordable and efficient healthcare. Our conversation drifted into us venting about what we each would do if we could change the world in one day to make healthcare better in this country.

COVID-19 has exposed the inefficiencies, inequities, lack of effectiveness, backwardness, and outdated processes and systems in our society. It has shown us just how many things in our society related to physical and mental health are just wrong.

EDUCATION

The first thing that I would do is totally overhaul our educational system.

To improve our current and future society, we have to start with our children. We need to make education the best we can provide for all children, despite what background they may come from or how much money their parents may or may not have. We need to overhaul our public-school system such that there is much less need for private and charter schools where people feel they can provide a better education for their children. Many people choose to send their children (with great sacrifice for many) to school outside of their local school system because they feel their public school system is sub-optimal. We need to overhaul school buildings to be outfitted with the most up-to-date equipment that is optimal for learning.

Those who educate children are really the backbone of our society because they form and shape our children into the adults and parents that we have in the future. I think we need to pay teachers, educators, and everyone involved in educating our children much more money so we can garner the best teachers which would offer an incentive for more people to become educators of young children. This would contribute to elevating teachers to a much higher status in our society.

Education with a focus on critical thinking and providing the foundation for young people to obtain marketable skills with vocational training, college preparation and/or entrepreneurial skills will make children better prepared to be independent and contribute to the world in the future.

HEALTH

We need to abolish health insurance being tied to employment. I think we need to totally overhaul our health system and illuminate private and commercial insurances and the medical industries that drive up costs of healthcare. I think these industries can be repurposed to do something else that will be beneficial to our society, keeping in mind that we need to remove the large profit that is built into our healthcare industry. Our health care is costing us too much and what we are paying is not sustainable. We have too many middle industries in our healthcare system. I think we need to model our healthcare system to be what universal healthcare actually means. We already have Medicare and Medicaid, which is almost universal healthcare already. So why not expand it and call it one name for everyone? Healthcare should be a right and not a privilege and should not be dependent on who you are and where you work. I think that people who still want to have their own private health insurance and who want to use a concierge-style healthcare can still be able to do that if they want to.

Other places in the world have converted to a more universal health care for all and I think we can provide this for everyone in the country with the resources that we have such that rationing of health care will not be necessary. I think our healthcare system overhaul has not happened because we have a minority of people who are benefiting financially from keeping things the way that they are: Unbalance, outdated educational system, outdated economy relying on outdated or obsolete industries that don't require the labor skills, large unskilled labor force languishing in our cities and rural areas, poor transportation system, relying on slow trains and cars, not allowing for access to goods and services, relying on employer-based health care, which keeps healthcare costs high. The pandemic has shown us that employer-based healthcare is useless when so many people in the country cannot work or should not be at work because of an infectious disease pandemic.

Everyone should be wearing a mask when they come out of their home. Full stop. We need a national plan that is targeted, efficient, comprehensive, and based on science to do COVID 19 testing and contact tracing to help decrease the transmission of the virus. We also need a national plan to encourage everyone to get vaccinated against COVID 19. In March of 2020, the healthcare community had to "stop and turn on a dime" to coordinate and provide care and testing for our patients in a disjointed way, because we had little to no guidance from the federal government to assist us. Many large institutions initially developed their own COVID 19 testing procedures because we could not wait for government assistance, while patients are presenting symptoms and serious illness from COVID 19. Initially, COVID 19 testing and then vaccination availability was too dependent on what city, county, and/or state you lived in. It should not matter where you reside whether you have access to COVID 19 testing, how long you have to wait for testing, how long you have to wait for your results, and how easy it is for you to get a COVID 19 vaccine. This global pandemic has proven to me definitively that we need more standardized, readily available universal health care.

MENTAL HEALTH AND PUBLIC SAFETY

We need to transform our system of public safety approaches with respect to community policing. This means that we must do a better job of managing our social and educational issues because criminal activity and interpersonal violence are often a consequence of our poor educational system, poor healthcare, poor support of people with mental health issues. Domestic violence and our other social ills are consequences of the failings in our society that lead to individual and collective behaviors that lead to law enforcement calls. We need to greatly invest in comprehensive and readily accessible behavioral/mental health and social work services for our country such that law enforcement does not need to be involved at all in these types of community calls for help and assistance. In addition, it seems that law enforcement officers who respond to community calls need to have training to de-escalate conflict and be held accountable if they do not. Anytime you have a law enforcement person that is called to a community scene with a gun, you are adding fuel to a fire, which could lead to a bad outcome. I think we need to pay our law enforcement officials more money, just like we need to pay our teachers more. By doing this, we can improve the quality of the pool of people who choose to do law enforcement. By transforming how we provide community assistance for mental health crises, law enforcement that carry guns will no longer need to be involved in these situations.

Criminalizing personal recreational cannabis use is futile and serves no purpose, other than to keep people unnecessarily engaged in our antiquated criminal justice system. Decriminalizing cannabis use will stop a lot of "crime" and violence related to this underground industry and the need for policing behavior related to the sale of marijuana. I think marijuana needs to be decriminalized on the national level and all state levels. As a physician, I think that cigarette smoking and alcohol use have always been a much greater risk to health and disease —greater than marijuana is. We are finding more and more ways of harnessing the medical benefits of cannabis.

I think that if we improve the daily lives (health, socially, economically) of the people in the country, we can eliminate the need for people to use drugs to escape from their life status. People often have used mind-altering substances because they are trying to evade the psychic stress from daily toxic environments. I think a lot of us become disappointed and resign to despair and use lots of substances and maladaptive behaviors. We use/abuse mind-altering and illicit drugs, food, sex, alcohol and prescription drugs to provide euphoria, no matter how temporary, to avoid psychological stress that has overwhelmed our lives.

ECONOMY/FOOD ECONOMY

It is often said that you can see what a person's values are by how they spend their money. If we look at what we spend money on, individually and collectively as a country, it is obvious that our focus is upside down.

We need to reinvent and re-imagine our economy and eliminate outdated industries in the food supply chain. And while they provide jobs and a living wage, they are now outdated and obsolete. Our focus should shift to new industries, products, and markets, focusing on helping our climate and changing how we think about growing food and food distribution. This includes totally overhauling how we eat, what we eat, and how we farm. Too much corn is being grown, along with raising too much beef. Our surplus of corn and starches has contributed to an excess of sugar in grocery store products. In addition to this, our habit of eating products from cows (beef, milk, cheese) has contributed to our obesity, cancer, and cardiovascular morbidity and mortality in this country.

We need to focus our thinking toward eating more vegetables and fruit and making sure that all neighborhoods have gardens, farms, and stores that allow access to fresh fruits and vegetables to be convenient and affordable to everyone.

Specifically, we have too much starch and sugar in our diet. Unfortunately, this goes hand-in-hand with improving our climate as we cannot grow the appropriate foods without having a climate that supports it. Sadly, many of the fruits and vegetables that we get from environments south of the United States are suffering from droughts and that is causing huge economic and population shifts that are affecting us. Our health and the food that we have available to us is impacted by climate change and political strife in other parts of the world.

The improvement in our collective nutrition should be considered by being mindful of what we all should be eating, what food we should be importing, and what we should grow to sell to others around the world.

INFRASTRUCTURE

In looking at our transportation system, I'd recommend huge improvements in how we move from place to place to go about our daily lives. We need to invest in high-speed trains which would greatly facilitate improvement in air and environmental pollution and traffic dilemmas in our large, overpopulated cities and allow more people to be able to live in more rural, less populated areas, while still having access to services that are available in large cities. With less reliance on personal cars, we can use more efficient public transportation and expand services that we all need to less populated areas such that more people have access to the things that we all need for daily living (food, healthcare, government services, broadband, etc.) and more people will be willing to move out of congested areas and still have access to employment, the ability to make a living, services, and products.

LABOR

Paying people to learn new skills would be one way to advance our labor force to be able to expand our economy to include new industries that address the needs of the current era and provide new jobs, careers and self-employment for people who will not be going back to their old form of employment. I believe that providing financial support to enable people to stay at home and prevent the transmission of the virus responsible for this global pandemic is a good idea. This means that businesses also need to be supported in such a way that it compensates for some of the losses that are occurring because people are not coming out in the community as much, utilizing these businesses in a customary way. Using money to support businesses to transform themselves to a new way of doing things would be useful as the world is changing to a "new normal."

And lastly, we need to get rid of the electoral college. It is outdated and unnecessary. I do not think it ever was necessary. We need one person, one vote, for all elections.

Appendix

ADVANCED DIRECTIVES

It is not pleasant to think about medical choices that you may have to make if you have a serious medical illness. However, we all need to think about what we want to do with our own care if we are temporarily or permanently incapacitated. This is called Advance Care Planning. Readily available forms of Advanced Directives are the MOLST (Medical Orders for Life-Sustaining Treatment) form and Five Wishes.

- https://molst.org/
- https://fivewishes.org/
- https://www.nia.nih.gov/health/advance-care-plan ning-health-care-directives

Advanced Directives are documentation of what you want to have done and who you want to make decisions for you in the event you cannot make decisions for yourself and/or you cannot communicate with a doctor and/or the team taking care of you.

Advanced Directives include two components:

- Living Will: What you want done in the event you cannot make medical decisions for yourself
- Durable Power of Attorney for Health Care: Who you want to make medical decisions for you in the event you cannot make medical decisions for yourself

We often think of Advanced Directives in terms of making end of life decisions in older persons, but in fact it is just as important for younger persons to have Advanced Directives and discuss end of life decisions because younger persons are more likely to have sudden illness (as opposed to a prolonged and/or chronic illness) such that they may not be able to ever communicate their wishes.

Sometimes the person closest to you is not the best person to carry out your wishes. Make sure that the Living Will is reviewed with the person that is being designated to make sure they can carry out these directives or wishes that are documented if the time comes. Advance Directives are also very important because at those times when you may become critically ill, family and friends "come out of the woodwork" and can try to make decisions for you. It is best to have wishes written down so they are respected and carried out as is desired. In addition, it is more comforting for your designated Health Care Power of Attorney to handle your affairs, as they will already be familiar with your wishes.

POWER OF ATTORNEY FOR HEALTH CARE AND LIVING WILL

This form is a combined Durable Power of Attorney for health care and a Living Will. With this form, you can name someone to make medical decisions for you, if in the future you're unable to make those decisions yourself.

You can also say what medical treatments you want and what medical treatments you don't want, if in the future, you're unable to make your wishes known.

You may change or cancel this document at any time.

Before you do Advanced Directives, talk to the person you want to name, to make sure that he/she understands your wishes and is willing to take the responsibility.

Give copies to your doctor, your nurse, the person you name to make your medical decisions for you, people in your family and anyone else who might be involved in your care. Discuss your Advance Directive with them.

- Advance directive: A written document (form) that tells what a person wants or doesn't want if he/she in the future can't make his/her wishes known about medical treatment.
- Artificial nutrition and hydration: When food and water are fed to a person through a tube.
- Autopsy: An examination done on a dead body to find the cause of death.
- Comfort care: Care that helps to keep a person comfortable but doesn't make him/her get well. Bathing, turning and keeping a person's lips moist are types of comfort care.
- CPR (cardiopulmonary resuscitation): Treatment to try to restart a person's breathing or heartbeat. CPR may be done by pushing on the chest, by putting a tube down the throat or by other treatment.
- Durable power of attorney for health care: An advance directive that names someone to make medical decisions

for a person if in the future he/she can't make his/her own medical decisions.

- Living will: An advance directive that tells what medical treatment a person does or doesn't want if he/she is not able to make his/her wishes known.

- Organ and tissue donation: When a person permits his/her organs (such as the eyes or kidneys) and other parts of the body (such as the skin) to be removed after death to be transplanted for use by another person or to be used for experimental purposes. Donating physical remains for academic study at a medical school is also a common choice.

- Life-sustaining treatment: Any medical treatment that is used to keep a person from dying. A breathing machine, CPR, artificial nutrition, antibiotics and hydration are examples of life-sustaining treatments.

- Persistent vegetative state: When a person is unconscious with no hope of regaining consciousness even with medical treatment. The body may move and the eyes may be open, but as far as anyone can tell, the person can't think or respond.

- Terminal condition: An ongoing condition caused by injury or illness that has no cure and from which doctors expect the person to die even with medical treatment. Life-sustaining treatments will only prolong the dying process if the person is suffering from a terminal condition.

COVID 19 AND TELEMEDICINE

This book gives my perspective on how patients can help their doctor provide them better care. The COVID 19 pandemic has changed how we deliver care by adding another dimension to delivering care on a broad scale. For those physicians who were reluctant to deliver care by telemedicine, the COVID 19 pandemic immediately instituted that option, probably forever, and there was no time for resistance. People were getting too sick too fast for physician resistance to the change.

In order to continue to deliver care, physicians, health care providers, doctor's offices, hospitals, home care agencies, nursing, long-term care, and rehab facilities, physical therapy facilities, outpatient labs, and radiology facilities and health care systems had to immediately shift procedures.

In the outpatient setting:

- Totally shift from seeing all patients in person to seeing most patients remotely, except for when absolutely needed to be seen face-to-face for at least 3 months (from March 2020 to the end of June 2020 at least) until we could slowly begin to bring patients into office.
- When we began seeing patients in the outpatient setting, we could not see the same volume of patients because of the disinfection and safety precautions that needed to be done in common spaces and patient exam rooms. Some offices could only see patients in the office one at a time. This meant that many patients could not be seen face-to-face as they wanted, when they wanted.
- There were increased staff responsibilities and duties with the same or fewer number of people to carry out the duties.

- Patient volume in the office was limited by staffing capacity for patient care, physical distancing, office space and exam room disinfection, leaving exam rooms dormant for a specified time after disinfection, trying not to become ill ourselves while maintaining social distancing from each other and wearing personal protective equipment.
- We were not in the office every day and were working remotely to provide care when physical office capacity restrictions did not allow for all staff to be in the office at the same time as before. Many office functions that we all took for granted became delayed and patients could not have the same level of service we used to provide.
- Office entrance infectious disease safety screening had to be done online and often rechecked with each patient upon arrival to the office.
- Only the patient was allowed into the office and in the exam room. Family members could no longer accompany the patient, unless the patient could not function during the visit on their own, without having someone with them.

What has been surprising to me, as we have been forced into immediately using telemedicine to deliver healthcare, is how resistant patients were to the change.

The technology to do telemedicine and video visits has been around for a long time. Technically, all that it takes is internet/Wi-Fi access and a device with a camera and a speaker. Unfortunately, access to this basic technology is not uniformly available to everyone.

But despite this societal failure, the medical community that provides face-to-face care with patients has been begging to be able to use this technology to deliver care for at least ten to fifteen years. However, the insurance industry, including Medicare and Medicaid, has not agreed to pay for it on a widespread basis. This indicates that there hasn't been enough emphasis on developing telemedicine software applications, enhancing cybersecurity measures, ensuring widespread broadband access, and providing personal devices to everyone.

Kaiser, on the other hand, because they are self-insured by the employers who contract for health services for their employees, has been using telemedicine since the late 1990's. Commercial insurance companies have been increasingly using telemedicine for their members, but this requires you get healthcare through your commercial insurance company from a remote doctor, NP (nurse practitioner) or PA (physician assistant) who does not know your medical history longitudinally. These medical encounters with a medical provider that does not see you on a regular basis are useful for non-serious medical conditions. The COVID-19 pandemic has forced commercial insurance companies and Medicare/Medicaid to now pay for telemedicine visits.

- https://mhealthintelligence.com/news/the-history-of-remote-monitoring-telemedicine-technology
- https://www.ncbi.nlm.nih.gov/books/NBK207141/

I remember that when the state of Maryland stay at home order was instituted on March 9, 2020, we were doing video visits within seven days at my large medical institution. But smaller institutions, groups and private practices were less able to shift so quickly to telemedicine to keep up with the pace of the raging viral pandemic stressors and restrictions that were placed on the ability to deliver healthcare. Fortunately, at my institution, we were already primed to start doing video visits anyway on our own just prior to that week in March 2020.

Much of what I do as an Internal Medicine physician is cognitive and does not require me to be in the same room as the patient. In primary care, much, if not most, of the delivery of their healthcare happens before, after, and in between their face-to-face office visits.

The face-to-face visit is often used to review what has happened with the patient in between visits.

Outside of a face-to-face visit, we provide services including but not limited to:

- Initiate and respond to telephone calls providing medical advice
- Reviewing charts in preparation for patient visits
- Post-visit patient chart documentation
- Review test results and communicate and/or coordinate test result communication to patients (phone, patient portal, letters).
- Prescribe and refill medications
- Sign orders for medications, home care, durable medical equipment
- Sign orders for home health care
- Respond to patient portal messages
- Order preventive health testing, diagnostic testing, lab orders
- Review patient portal entered home monitoring values (blood pressure, blood glucose, home INR monitoring)
- Review internal and external medical records, when received on paper and electronically

- Review and respond to internal and external documents from ED and urgent care visits
- Review and respond to internal and physician and provider communication for coordination of care (home care providers, radiologists, specialists, nurses)
- Reviewing patient charts to coordinate preventive care scheduling of testing, appointments, chronic disease management (immunizations, breast cancer screening, colon cancer screening, diabetic eye care, diabetic foot care, etc.)
- Reviewing patient lists for outreach for missed appointments, canceled appointments, preventive care gap outreach, chronic disease management outreach

I have found many positive aspects to delivering care by telemedicine in the primary care setting. With a video visit, facial expression and body language can still be an integral part of the interaction between me and the patient. Wearing masks during face-to-face visits led to the loss of the ability to see facial expressions during the visit, and I felt an immediate change and disorientation in the interactions that I was having with my patients due to not being able to see their reactions and them not being able to see mine. I've had to adjust my speech and language cues, body language, how I stand and sit in the exam room, speaking tone and how I ask and respond to questions due to wearing masks and social distancing during the face-to-face patient encounter.

A video visit has the advantage of the patient being seen in their home environment with family members involved in the visit. Starting in 2020 and extending into the first half of 2021, only the adult patient was allowed in the patient care area, unless they needed to be accompanied by another adult. I have used tele-medicine visits to travel through the patient's kitchen and pantry and have meaningful discussions about what food they should and should not be eating, helping them read food labels to make healthier food choices.

Telemedicine has been very useful for older patients that are frail and have difficulty leaving the home to come to the office, and it is also very useful for communicating with family members during the video visit, as the currently available platforms allow multiple people, along with the patient, to participate in the vis-it when desired or needed. For my senior patients, the video visit allowed me to talk to everyone in the house who was involved in the patients' care, and I was able to communicate with more of the family than the one person who typically came with the pa-tient's face-to-face office visits prior to the pandemic. Extended family members are very helpful with providing care to older pa-tients to make sure that orders are carried out, referrals are being done, medications are being taken and to supervise the patient's eating habits in-between visits.

I have found that I have been able to deliver better care by tele-medicine to patients who have a caregiver or care partner because I have been able to more consistently have caregivers be involved in-patient visits when the caregiver cannot come to the office with the patient. As mentioned earlier, video visits typically require a desktop, laptop, tablet or at least a smartphone with a camera and audio. Many older patients only have "flip phones" that are not amenable to doing a video visit. This required family members to get involved in care to facilitate the visits which led to more lasting family involvement in care that is enduring in 2021.

Telemedicine visits are excellent to use to quickly evaluate and treat minor medical conditions, like upper respiratory symptoms, musculoskeletal conditions, and dermatologic conditions, and to deliver chronic disease management care, without a face-to-face visit. This care is delivered very efficiently without the patient having to change their day to accommodate for travel time in order to be seen. Video visits are an efficient way to address urgent issues that may be new or exacerbations of chronic medical conditions. In Internal Medicine/primary care, the most important part of addressing an issue with a patient is not just about what I can physically touch and see, but it is about listening to the patient, taking a history of the symptoms along with reviewing their overall medical history to put the pieces of the puzzle together to address the issues for the visit.

A video visit prevents the limitation of geography and location when delivering healthcare, eliminating the challenge of traveling to a building to receive care and the ability to receive care at home when transportation, physical and medical conditions pose challenges to being able to come to a doctor's office. Video visits allow for more flexible scheduling for urgent issues and it allows me to have flexible scheduling to talk to family members during a video when they cannot come with the patient. Telemedicine allows us to deliver healthcare that is impactful and meaningful without a face-to-face visit.

Transitioning to doing video visits was met with many resistant and frankly belligerent patients who refused to engage in video visits and delayed their care during 2020. I had patients absolutely refuse to engage in this technology after trying to do outreach to them with telephone calls, patient portal messages, and written letters sent to their homes.

Many patients had difficulty stepping out of their comfort zone and re-imagining the concept of what healthcare is, how it should be delivered and what kind of healthcare delivery they will accept as legitimate. It has been a challenge over the last year to get patients to change their perspective on how they receive their health care.

Fortunately, many patients have tried and had successful video visits by now, even the most reluctant ones. I think my patients have become more comfortable with this form of healthcare delivery over the last 24 months because they have been able to still have meaningful communication with their doctor, especially with respect to chronic disease management.

It has been very challenging trying to deliver the same quality health care, while trying to appreciate and respond to the perception of healthcare delivery from the patient's perspective. The goal was to have patients still feel satisfied with their health care. It was difficult to get people to shift their understanding of receiving healthcare such that they were comfortable that I could manage many of their concerns and chronic conditions without us being in the same room. Over the last 12 months, patients have had video visits and have returned to coming into the office and have realized that much of what we do face-to-face was being accomplished in the video visit.

Office visits for blood pressure management are important for obvious reasons but also to have patients bring in their blood pressure machine to be checked for proper use and accuracy is also key. But after that, home blood pressure monitoring is much more important to see what the daily blood pressure pattern is.

I have encouraged patients to try to change their way of thinking about how they receive care, because video visits are here to stay and have been an important addition to allow more variability in healthcare delivery by removing limitations of location and the need for travel time to and from doctors' offices.

Video visits have been useful for people who have healthcare conditions that make it unsafe for them to come to a doctor's office or medical facility due to concerns of COVID-19 exposure and infection. Many of these patients have reasons not to come to a medical facility long prior to the pandemic.

The use of the video visit forced many people to sign up for the patient portal. I had many patients who never reviewed all of the available information in the patient portal and verbalized how surprised they were about how much content was available to help manage and improve their health. The pandemic has pushed patients to use technology and many have embraced or at least have accepted the transition. We've had a great increase in the number of patients using the EMR and/or patient portals to communicate with the healthcare delivery team (doctor, nurses, pharmacies) and to use this technology to manage their own care (prescription refills, reviewing test results, reviewing preventive care gaps).

For the moment, our schedules have been adjusted to allow more in-office visits. Many patients are still concerned about coming into medical facilities. Video visits are now a permanent aspect of our daily and weekly schedules, which does not negate or eliminate the in-person visit.

TELEMEDICINE EXAM

In 2020, physicians learned very quickly how to modify our interaction with patients to perform, often with assistance of the patient document examination and findings, video encounters and virtual encounters and interactions with the patients.

Here are some medical vitals/actions/observations that can be done without coming into the medical office:

VITAL SIGNS

You can provide your weight, blood pressure, pulse oxygen saturation, temperature to be evaluated by your doctor. Many patients now have scales, blood pressure monitors, pulse oximeters, and thermometers in their homes to check weight, blood pressure pulse, oxygen saturation, and temperature. The technology for digital remote monitoring devices will likely be used in a more widespread fashion within the next 1-5 years I expect.

GENERAL/PSYCHIATRIC

Your general appearance can be observed by your doctor. Any distress and agitation you are having can be observed. Your mental status and mood can be evaluated.

RESPIRATORY

Your doctor can observe your breathing, see any coughing, look at your breathing rate, look at you while you are taking a deep breath, and observe and listen for wheezing and fast breathing, abnormal breathing sounds.

Use of digital stethoscopes to hear breath sounds will likely be used clinically or more widespread in the future.

GASTROINTESTINAL

Your doctor can see abdominal distension and abdominal firmness on camera, and you can push on your abdomen to show your doctor where you have belly pain. Use of digital stethoscopes to hear bowel sounds will likely be used clinically or more widespread in the future.

EAR, NOSE, MOUTH, AND THROAT

- Throat and neck swelling can be observed by your doctor. Your head can be observed.
- Inside of the mouth, tongue, back of throat and lips can be looked at. Nasal drainage can be seen.
- You can assist with sinus evaluation on the face.
- Use of digital otoscopes will likely be used clinically or more widespread in the future.

SKIN

Your doctor can see bruising, rashes and many skin changes easily by video. Patients often send pictures of external findings on the body using the patient portal and these images can be incorporated in the video visit.

HEART

Your doctor can see swelling of neck veins. Your doctor can instruct you how to check your pulse. You can press your thumb into your legs to show your doctor any leg swelling, and you can feel coolness in the legs to report to your doctor. You can show any discoloration of the leg.

Use of digital stethoscopes to hear heart sounds will likely be used clinically or more widespread in the future.

NERVES AND BRAIN

Your doctor can see face and tongue movements for evidence of neurologic abnormalities. Basic vision, hearing, and sense of smell can be assessed by your doctor. Your doctor can observe color of the eyes, status of eyelids, eye movements and eye discharge. You can use a flashlight to evaluate pupil movement of your eyes. Your doctor can have you do maneuvers to check your speech, walking, raising arms and legs, standing from a seated position. Any tremors you may have can be observed. Basic neurologic movements can be evaluated in your face, arms, and legs. Your walking/gait can be observed. Joint range of motion can be observed.

LYMPH NODES
You can be instructed on how to feel your neck for enlarged lymph nodes with visualization by the doctor.

MUSCULAR
Neck pain with rotation can be observed. Fingers and toes can be observed. Joint movements (neck, back, shoulder, elbow, knees, wrists, fingers, ankle) and pain with joint movements can be seen by your doctor.

EXTERNAL GENITALIA
External skin and scrotum can be seen by your doctor, and you can provide images that can be reviewed by your doctor.

Here are resources for more information about Telemedicine:

- https://www.ncbi.nlm.nih.gov/pmc/articles/PMC7368154/
- https://telehealth.hhs.gov/providers/preparing-patients-for-telehealth/telehealth-physical-exam

Resources

INTRODUCTION

https://time.com/6279937/
us-health-care-system-attitudes/

https://health.usnews.com/
health-care/top-doctors/articles/primary-care-
experiences-survey-report#:~:text=25%25%20
said%20they%20don't,others%20during%20
a%20PCP%20visit

https://www.cnn.com/2023/01/31/health/
us-health-care-spending-global-perspective/
index.html

https://www.ama-assn.org/press-center/press-releases/ama-president-sounds-alarm-national-physician-shortage

CHAPTER FIVE

https://www.uspreventiveservicestaskforce.org/uspstf

https://www.choosingwisely.org/our-mission/history/

https://www.cdc.gov/mmwr/volumes/68/wr/mm6832a3.htm

https://www.cdc.gov/vaccines/hcp/acip-recs/vacc-specific/pneumo.html

https://www.uspreventiveservicestaskforce.
org/uspstf/recommendation/
hepatitis-c-screening

https://www.uspreventiveservicestaskforce.
org/uspstf/recommendation/
colorectal-cancer-screening

https://www.cdc.gov/vaccines/hcp/acip-recs/
vacc-specific/shingles.html

https://www.uspreventiveservicestaskforce.
org/uspstf/recommendation/
osteoporosis-screening

https://www.cancer.org/cancer/lung-cancer/
detection-diagnosis-staging/detection.html

https://www.cancer.org/cancer/prostate-
cancer/detection-diagnosis-staging/
acs-recommendations.html

https://www.uspreventiveservicestaskforce.org/uspstf/recommendation/prostate-cancer-screening

https://www.uptodate.com/contents/prostate-cancer-screening-beyond-the-basics?topicRef=7567&source=see_link

CHAPTER SIX

https://www.healthgrades.com/right-care/sexual-health/9-questions-to-ask-about-your-partners-sexual-history

https://www.plannedparenthood.org/learn/stds-hiv-safer-sex/get-tested/how-do-i-talk-my-partner-about-std-testing

https://www.cdc.gov/flu/about/index.htmlhttps://www.cdc.gov/mmwr/volumes/69/rr/rr6908a1.htm

https://wwwnc.cdc.gov/travel/destinations/list

https://www.healthit.gov/topic/
patient-access-health-records/
patient-access-health-records

https://www.healthit.gov/curesrule/
overview/about-oncs-cures-act-final-rule

CHAPTER ELEVEN

https://www.choosingwisely.org/
our-mission/history/

CHAPTER THIRTEEN

https://www.cancer.org/healthy/
find-cancer-early/american-cancer-society-
guidelines-for-the-early-detection-of-cancer.
html

https://www.komen.org/breast-
cancer/screening/when-to-screen/
average-risk-women/

https://www.touch4life.org/

CHAPTER SIXTEEN

https://www.healthline.com/health/
cholesterol/advanced-cholesterol-test

https://www.healthline.com/health/
heart-disease/coronary-calcium-score

CHAPTER SEVENTEEN

https://www.validatebp.org/

https://www.healthline.com/health/
how-to-check-blood-pressure-by-hand

CHAPTER NINETEEN

https://www.
hamiltonhealthsciences.ca/share/
ergonomics-tips-for-working-remotely/

https://www.publichealthdegrees.org/
resources/how-to-create-work-from-home-
set-up/

https://www.uhs.wisc.edu/wp-content/
uploads/2020/03/Remote-Workspace-
Ergonomics-3-18-20.pdf

CHAPTER TWENTY-ONE

https://www.cdc.gov/high-blood-pressure/about/?CDC_AAref_Val=https://www.cdc.gov/bloodpressure/about.htm

https://www.ncbi.nlm.nih.gov/pmc/articles/PMC4473614/

CHAPTER TWENTY-TWO

https://www.ahajournals.org/doi/10.1161/CIR.0000000000000678?url_ver=Z39.88-2003&rfr_id=ori:rid:crossref.org&rfr_dat=cr_pub%3dpubmed

https://www.healthline.com/health/stroke/stroke-screening

https://www.healthline.com/health/cholesterol-test

https://internal.mesa-nhlbi.org/about/overview

https://www.healthline.com/health/heart-disease/coronary-calcium-score

https://www.healthline.com/health/cholesterol/advanced-cholesterol-test

https://www.youtube.com/watch?v=0zkLGawMtwc

https://www.healthline.com/health/carotid-duplex

CHAPTER TWENTY-THREE

https://www.cdc.gov/obesity/php/data-research/adult-obesity-facts.html?CDC_AAref_Val=https://www.cdc.gov/obesity/data/adult.html

CHAPTER TWENTY-FOUR

https://www.healthline.com/nutrition/intermittent-fasting-side-effects

CHAPTER TWENTY-FIVE

https://www.healthline.com/nutrition/optimize-omega-6-omega-3-ratio#TOC_TITLE_HDR_5

READING FOOD LABELS:

https://www.fda.gov/food/nutrition-facts-label/how-understand-and-use-nutrition-facts-label

https://www.heart.org/en/healthy-living/ healthy-eating/eat-smart/nutrition-basics/ understanding-food-nutrition-labels

https://www.nia.nih.gov/health/how-read-food-and-beverage-labels

https://www.healthline.com/nutrition/ how-to-read-food-labels

CHAPTER TWENTY-SEVEN

https://www.sugarnutritionresource.org/ the-basics/sugars-on-food-labels

https://sugarscience.ucsf.edu/hidden-in-plain-sight/#.YOtL8nlKiUk

https://www.healthline.com/nutrition/ too-much-sugar

https://www.healthline.com/nutrition/
how-much-sugar-per-day

CHAPTER TWENTY-EIGHT

https://www.health.harvard.edu/
staying-healthy/the-truth-about-metabolism

https://www.healthline.com/health/
exercise-fitness/ideal-body-fat-percentage

https://www.healthline.com/nutrition/
ways-to-measure-body-fat

https://www.xyngular.com/en/blog/
how-to-measure-weight-loss-without-a-scale/

https://www.cosmed.com/en/contact-us/
test-site-locator

https://www.cdc.gov/healthyweight/
assessing/bmi/adult_bmi/english_bmi_
calculator/bmi_caculator.html

https://www.mayoclinicproceedings.org/
article/S0025-6196(18)30807-3/fulltext

CHAPTER THIRTY-SIX

https://www.habibibodysport.com/

CHAPTER THIRTY-EIGHT

https://www.sleepfoundation.
org/insomnia/treatment/
cognitive-behavioral-therapy-insomnia

https://stanfordhealthcare.org/
medical-treatments/c/cognitive-
behavioral-therapy-insomnia/procedures/
stimulus-control.html

APPENDIX

ADVANCED DIRECTIVES

https://molst.org/

https://fivewishes.org/

https://www.nia.nih.gov/health/
advance-care-planning-health-care-directives

COVID 19 AND TELEMEDICINE

https://mhealthintelligence.com/news/
the-history-of-remote-monitoring-
telemedicine-technology

https://www.ncbi.nlm.nih.gov/books/
NBK207141/

https://www.ncbi.nlm.nih.gov/pmc/articles/PMC7368154/

https://telehealth.hhs.gov/providers/preparing-patients-for-telehealth/telehealth-physical-exam

ARTICLES AND BOOKS REGARDING BIAS IN CLINICAL CARE GUIDELINES

https://www.acoi.org/sites/default/files/uploads/advocacy/AOA%20and%20ACOI%20Comment%20AHRQ%20Clinical%20Algorithms%20RFI_05042021_FINAL.pdf

https://journalofethics.ama-assn.org/article/race-discrimination-and-cardiovascular-disease/2014-06

https://jamanetwork.com/journals/jamacardiology/fullarticle/2492412

https://www.ccjm.org/content/90/11/685

https://ucheblackstock.com/

Acknowledgements

I WOULD LIKE TO THANK MY MOTHER, GRANDMOTHER, siblings, my husband and my many patients who have given me encouragement and support along my journey.

I would also like to thank Regina Gill, MS, RD, LDN who gave an invaluable contribution to the nutrition advice provided in this book.

About the Author

D R. COE IS A PRACTICING INTERNIST/PRIMARY CARE physician experienced with taking care of adult patients in the outpatient, nursing home and hospital setting. She has practiced in private practice and group practice settings, including academic practices teaching medical students and residents. She has also served on a medical school admission committee as well. She has spent her career seeing patients in the specialty of Internal Medicine for over 20 years and has worked in academic settings teaching medical students and medical residents with direct patient care in clinical medical school faculty positions. She has done numerous speaking engagements (in person, radio, webinars) for laypersons, colleagues and corporate audiences over the course of her career about various topics, including informing audiences about preventive health, chronic disease management and most recently, COVID 19. She has written many health and wellness articles in print and online for public facing professional, community and hospital platforms.

She received a BA in Human Biology from Stanford University, a medical degree from the Howard University College of Medicine and an MBA from Baldwin Wallace College in Ohio.

WEBSITE

https://besthealthforyourlife.com/

LINKEDIN

www.linkedin.com/in/docbbesthealth4life

FACEBOOK

Best Health For Your Life Consulting LLC

INSTAGRAM

@docb_besthealth4life

X

docB_besthealth4life

www.ingramcontent.com/pod-product-compliance
Lightning Source LLC
Chambersburg PA
CBHW052109030426
42335CB00025B/2910